16th International Conference on

Production Diseases in Farm Animals

–

Book of abstracts

16th International Conference on

Production Diseases in Farm Animals

–

Book of abstracts

ICPD 2016

Wageningen, the Netherlands

20-23 June 2016

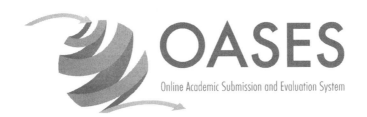

EAN: 9789086862856
e-EAN: 9789086868315
ISBN: 978-90-8686-285-6
e-ISBN: 978-90-8686-831-5
DOI: 10.3920/978-90-8686-831-5

First published, 2016

© Wageningen Academic Publishers
The Netherlands, 2016

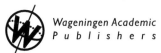

This work is subject to copyright. All rights are reserved, whether the whole or part of the material is concerned. Nothing from this publication may be translated, reproduced, stored in a computerised system or published in any form or in any manner, including electronic, mechanical, reprographic or photographic, without prior written permission from the publisher:
Wageningen Academic Publishers
P.O. Box 220
6700 AE Wageningen
The Netherlands
www.WageningenAcademic.com
copyright@WageningenAcademic.com

The individual contributions in this publication and any liabilities arising from them remain the responsibility of the authors.

The publisher is not responsible for possible damages, which could be a result of content derived from this publication.

Organising Committee

Bas Kemp	Wageningen UR, Adaptation Physiology Group
Wouter Hendriks	Wageningen UR, Animal Nutrition Group
Thomas Schonewille	Utrecht University, Faculty of Veterinary Medicine
Gert van Duinkerken	Wageningen UR Livestock Research
Ariëtte van Knegsel	Wageningen UR, Adaptation Physiology Group
Astrid de Greeff	Central Veterinary Institute of Wageningen UR
Roselinde Goselink	Wageningen UR Livestock Research

Scientific Committee

Christer Bergsten	Swedish University of Agricultural Sciences
Liesbeth Bolhuis	Wageningen UR, Adaptation Physiology Group
Henk Hogeveen	Wageningen UR, Business Economics Group
Josef Kamphues	University of Veterinary Medicine Hannover
Ilias Kyriazakis	Newcastle University
Matt Lucy	University of Missouri
David Renaudeau	INRA Rennes
Bas Rodenburg	Wageningen UR, Behavioural Ecology Group
Helga Sauerwein	University of Bonn
Hauke Smidt	Wageningen UR, Microbiology Group

Partners

Wageningen UR

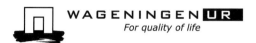

Utrecht University

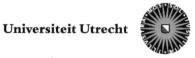

Diamond V

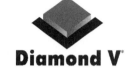

Hatchtech

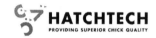

Zinpro

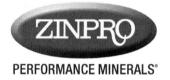

Contact

ICPD 2016
PO Box 338
6700 AH Wageningen
The Netherlands
icpd.2016@wur.nl
http://icpd2016.wur.nl

Welcome!

Dear Participants,

Welcome to the 16th International Conference on Production Diseases in Farm Animals!

The organising institutes Wageningen UR and Utrecht University, as well as their organising partners Diamond V, Hatchtech and Zinpro, are proud to have you as our guests.

The goal of the ICPD is to unite scientists from different disciplines and various countries to advance the study and understanding of health and disease in animals managed for food production. It has its roots in the study of metabolic and nutritional diseases affecting health and welfare of farm animals. The ICPD 2016 will provide the recent research results on those aspects in the different farm animal species.

Of course we would like to express our gratitude to all contributors of the ICPD 2016: the session chairs, the invited speakers, the presenting authors in the poster and theatre sessions and all delegates contributing to the conference.

We sincerely hope that this event will contribute to your expertise and ideas on important aspects of the animal production of the future. We gratefully acknowledge Diamond V, Hatchtech and Zinpro for their support in organizing this event.

The organising committee

Bas Kemp, Wouter Hendriks, Thomas Schonewille, Gert van Duinkerken,
Ariëtte van Knegsel, Astrid de Greeff and Roselinde Goselink

List of previous ICPDs

I.   **Urbana-Champaign, Illinois, 1968**

II.   **Reading, England, 1972**

III.   **Wageningen, The Netherlands, 1976**

IV.   **Munich, Germany, 1980**

V.   **Uppsala, Sweden, 1983**

VI.   **Belfast, Northern Ireland, 1986**

VII.   **Ithaca, New York, 1989**

VIII.   **Bern, Switzerland, 1992**

IX.   **Berlin, Germany, 1995**

X.   **Utrecht, The Netherlands, 1998**

XI.   **Copenhagen, Denmark, 2001**

XII.   **East Lansing, Michigan, 2004**

XIII.   **Leipzig, Germany, 2007**

XIV.   **Ghent, Belgium, 2010**

XV.   **Uppsala, Sweden, 2013**

XVI.   **Wageningen, The Netherlands, 2016**

General Information

Welcome reception

The welcome reception on **Monday 20 June** will be in Hotel de Wageningsche Berg.
Address: Generaal Foulkesweg 96, 6703 DS Wageningen
Phone: +31 317 495 911

Conference venue

The conference venue **from 21-23 June** is Hof van Wageningen, Hotel and Conference Centre.
Address: Lawickse Allee 9, 6701 AN Wageningen
Phone: +31 317 490 133

Conference rooms
Theatre presentations will be on the first floor in two rooms: "Ir Haakzaal" and "Kleine Veerzaal".
Poster presentations will be on the ground floor in "Wolfswaardzaal".
Coffee and lunch will be served on the ground floor in "Terraszaal".

Conference secretariat and upload room

Hotel de Wageningsche Berg
Monday 20 June   17.00-19.00

Hof van Wageningen, Hotel and Conference Centre
Room: "Bornzaal"
Tuesday 21 June   07.30-18.00
Wednesday 22 June   07.30-17.00
Thursday 23 June   07.30-17.00

Entrance tickets

Your name badge – received at the registration desk – is your admission to the scientific sessions, coffee, and lunches. It should be worn at all times at the conference venue.
If you have also booked for the social events (excursion to the animal facilities with dinner buffet 22 June (€15) and/or excursion to Burgers' Zoo with conference dinner 23 June (€50)), you have received those entrance tickets as well – please take them to the event.

Internet access

Wireless Internet access is available at the Hof van Wageningen Conference Centre.

Public transport

For information about public transport (bus, train) to get around Wageningen, please visit http://9292.nl/en.

Social events

Welcome reception

Monday 20 June, 17.00 - 19.00h

The registration and welcome reception will take place in Hotel de Wageningsche Berg, at walking distance (3 km) from the conference venue. Address: Generaal Foulkesweg 96, 6703 DS Wageningen.

Excursion to animal facilities

Wednesday 22 June, 16.30 - 20.00h

An excursion to the animal facilities CARUS will be combined with a dinner buffet at the Wageningen UR Campus.
Buses will transport you from the Hof van Wageningen Conference Centre to the Wageningen UR Campus (16.00h) and return around 20.00h.

Excursion to Burgers' Zoo

Thursday 23 June, 17.00 -23.30h

Buses will leave at 17.00h for an excursion to Burgers' Zoo in Arnhem. The excursion will start with an invited lecture of Dr. Constanze Mager, after which a short guided tour will be organised followed by the conference dinner. Buses will return to Wageningen from 22.00-23.30h.

Maps of Wageningen

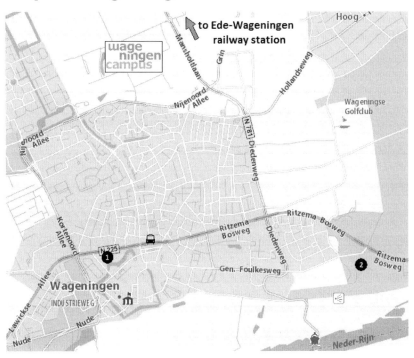

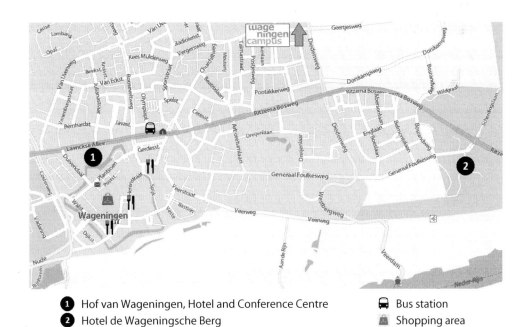

❶	Hof van Wageningen, Hotel and Conference Centre	🚌	Bus station
❷	Hotel de Wageningsche Berg	🛍	Shopping area
		🍴	Restaurants

Programme at a glance

Monday 20 June

17.00-19.00h   Welcome reception and registration

Location: Hotel de Wageningsche Berg, Generaal Foulkesweg 96, 6703 DS Wageningen.

Tuesday 21 June to Thursday 23 June

Location: Hof van Wageningen, Hotel and Conference Centre, Lawickse Allee 9,
          6701 AN Wageningen.

Tuesday 21 June *Registration from 7.30h*		Wednesday 22 June *Registration from 7.30h*	Thursday 23 June *Registration from 7.30h*	
8.30-9.00h **Opening**		8.30-10.15h **5 Adaptation to lactation** *Ir Haakzaal*	8.30-10.15h **8 PROHEALTH** *Ir Haakzaal*	8.30-10.15h **9 Reproduction** *Kleine Veerzaal*
9.00-10.30h **1 Locomotion** *Ir Haakzaal*	9.00-10.30h **2 Poultry** *Kleine Veerzaal*	10.15-10.45h Coffee break	10.15-10.45h Coffee break	
10.30-11.00h Coffee break		10.45-12.00h **5 Adaptation to lactation** *Ir Haakzaal*	10.45-12.00h **8 PROHEALTH** *Ir Haakzaal*	10.45-12.00h **9 Reproduction** *Kleine Veerzaal*
11.00-12.30h **1 Locomotion** *Ir Haakzaal*	11.00-12.30h **2 Poultry** *Kleine Veerzaal*	12.00-13.30h Lunch break **Poster session 5, 6, 7**	12.00-13.30h Lunch break **Poster session 8, 9, 10, 11**	
12.30-14.00h Lunch break **Poster session 1, 2, 3, 4**		13.30-15.15h **6 Economics of disease** *Ir Haakzaal*	13.30-15.00h **10 Welfare production trade-offs** *Ir Haakzaal*	
14.00-15.30h **3 Gut health** *Ir Haakzaal*	14.00-15.30h **4 Heat stress** *Kleine Veerzaal*	14.15-15.30h **7 Free com. I** *Kleine Veerzaal*	15.00-15.30h Coffee break	
15.30-16.00h Coffee break		15.30-16.00h Coffee break	15.30-17.00h **10 Welfare** *Ir Haakzaal*	15.30-17.00h **11 Free com. II** *Kleine Veerzaal*
16.00-17.15h **3 Gut health** *Ir Haakzaal*	16.00-17.15h **4 Heat stress** *Kleine Veerzaal*	16.00h bus transfer to Wageningen UR Campus		
		16.30-21.00h Excursion to research facilities CARUS	17.00h bus transfer to Burgers' Zoo Arnhem	
			18.00-23.30h Invited lecture Dr. Constanze Mager	
		Buffet at Campus	**Conference Dinner**	

Table of contents

Session 01. Locomotion disorders

Chairperson: Prof. Dr. Christer Bergsten, Swedish University of Agricultural Sciences
Date: 21 June – 9.00-12.30h
Location: Ir Haakzaal

Theatre Session 01

9.00h Early lameness detection, cow comfort and infectious lesion control: lessons from the UK 31
invited N. Bell

9.45h Gait cycle in dairy cows and its application to detect lameness 32
M. Alsaaod, T. Hausegger, R. Kredel and A. Steiner

10.00h Use of extended locomotor behavior characteristics for automated identification of lame dairy cows 33
G. Beer, M. Alsaaod, A. Starke, G. Regula-Schüpbach, H. Müller, P. Kohler and A. Steiner

10.15h Use of routine collected herd data to estimate claw health in dairy herds 34
H. Brouwer, T. Dijkstra, H. Worm, Y. Van Der Vorst and G. Van Schaik

10.30h Coffee break

11.00h Digital dermatitis in dairy cattle: infectivity of the different stages 35
F. Biemans, P. Bijma and M.C.M. De Jong

11.15h Prevalence, risk factors and bacterial species associated with non-healing white line disorders 36
E. Van Engelen, M. Gonggrijp, M. Holzhauer, A. Ten Wolthuis and A. Velthuis

11.30h Perceptions about the causes, treatment and prevention of lameness in a pasture-based dairy industry 37
J. Marchewka, J.F. Mee and L.A. Boyle

11.45h The effect of rubber-covered floors on gait and claw lesions in group-housed gestating sows 38
E.-J. Bos, D. Maes, M. Van Riet, S. Millet, B. Ampe, G. Janssens and F. Tuyttens

12.00h Physical exercise of dairy cows: effects of training on activity, lying behaviour and heart rate 39
W. Ouweltjes, G.P. Binnendijk and R.M.A. Goselink

12.15h Physical exercise of dairy cows: effects of training on energy balance   40
    R.M.A. Goselink, G.P. Binnendijk and W. Ouweltjes

Poster Session 01

Case report: leg lameness in gilts   41
    E. De Jong and P. Bonny

Effect of hydroxy-copper and -zinc and L-selenomethionine on claw health of sows   42
    A.B.J. Van Dalen and I. Eising

Mycoplasma arthritis outbreaks in dairy herds   43
    M. Holzhauer, R. Dijkman, E. Van Engelen, M.A. Gonggrijp and K. Junker

Quantification of extended characteristics of locomotor behavior in dairy cows   44
    M. Alsaaod, J. Niederhauser, G. Schüpbach-Regula, G. Beer and A. Steiner

Effectiveness of copper sulfate solutions in footbaths   45
    A. Prastiwi, Z. Okumus, A. Hayirli, D. Celebi, L. Yanmaz, E. Dogan and U. Ersoz

Session 02. Production diseases in poultry

Chairperson: Prof. Dr. Josef Kamphues, University of Veterinary Medicine Hannover
Date: 21 June – 9.00-12.30h
Location: Kleine Veerzaal

Theatre Session 02

9.00h The quality of light and its intensity in housing of poultry: potential effects
    on behavior   46
invited *R. Korbel*

9.45h New approaches in housing and management to improve foot pad health
    in fattening poultry   47
invited *I.C. De Jong and J. Van Harn*

10.30h Coffee break

11.00h Feather pecking and cannibalism in 107 organic laying hen flocks in 8
    European countries   48
    M. Bestman, C. Verwer, F. Smajlhodzic, J.L.T. Heerkens, L.K. Hinrichsen, C. Brenninkmeyer,
    V. Ferrante, A. Willet and S. Gunnarsson

11.15h Radiographic examination of deformities and fractures of keel bones in
    laying hens   49
    B.K. Eusemann, U. Baulain, L. Schrader and S. Petow

11.30h Nutritional dietary tools to reduce the incidence of fatty liver syndrome in
    laying hens   50
    A. Navarro-Villa, J. Mica, J. De Los Mozos and A.I. García-Ruiz

11.45h Hepatic lipidosis: histological and chemical characterization of healthy and
    diseased turkey livers   51
    D. Radko, R. Günther, A. Engels, C. Leibfacher and C. Visscher

12.00h Sharp decrease of AmpC-E. coli in a broiler parent stock flock   52
    M.A. Dame-Korevaar, E.A.J. Fischer, A. Van Essen-Zandbergen, K.T. Veldman,
    J.A. Stegeman, D.J. Mevius and J.A. Van Der Goot

12.15h Link between diet particle size, stomach morphology and incidence of
    cecal *Campylobacter* in broilers   53
    S.J. Sander, B. Üffing, M. Witte, A. Beineke, J. Verspohl and J. Kamphues

Poster Session 02

Finely ground soybean byproducts in broiler diets: performance, excreta quality
and foot pad health   54
    A. Heuermann, M. Kölln, T. Jackisch and J. Kamphues

A new floor design for housing fattening poultry to minimize animal's contact
with excreta   55
    C. Visscher and J. Kamphues

Effect of floor design in broiler housing on development of resistance in
commensal *Escherichia coli*   56
    B. Chuppava, B. Keller and C. Visscher

A byproduct of swine slaughtering in broiler diets: effect on performance and foot
pad health   57
    M. Kölln, A. Loi-Brügger and J. Kamphues

Session 03. Gut health and microbiota

Chairperson: Prof. Dr. Hauke Smidt, Wageningen UR
Date: 21 June – 14.00-17.15h
Location: Ir Haakzaal

Theatre Session 03

14.00h Enhancing gastrointestinal robustness to prevent major pig and poultry
    production diseases   58
    invited *O. Hojberg, N. Canibe, R.M. Engberg, B.B. Jensen and C. Lauridsen*

14.30h Nutritional modulation of the intestinal microbiota: host interplay in weaned pigs   59
invited R. Pieper

15.00h Neonatal development of the gut of broilers is influenced by genetics and
          management   60
          D. Schokker, A.J.M. Jansman, M.A. Smits and J.M.J. Rebel

15.15h Secondary plant compounds to reduce the use of antibiotics   61
          R. Aschenbroich and I. Heinzl

15.30h Coffee break

16.00h Epidemiology, pathogenicity and inhibition of APEC isolated from
          commercial broilers in Georgia, USA   62
          A. Wealleans, K. Gibbs, J. Benson, F. Delago, J. Lambrecht, M. Bernardeau and E. Galbraith

16.15h *In vitro* antimicrobial activity of cinnamaldehyde derivatives against the
          piglet gut microbiota   63
          C. Forte, E. Ruysbergh, A. Ovyn, S. De Smet, S. Mangelinckx and J. Michiels

16.30h The effects of medium chain fatty acids after maternal or neonatal
          administration to piglets   64
          A. De Greeff, J. Allaart, D. Schokker, C. De Bruijn, S.A. Vastenhouw, P. Roubos, M.A. Smits
          and J.M.J. Rebel

16.45h Effects of rye inclusion in diets on broiler performance, gut morphology
          and microbiota composition   65
          M.M. Van Krimpen, M. Torki, S. Borgijink, D. Schokker, S. Vastenhouw, F.M. De Bree,
          A. Bossers, T. Fabri, N. De Bruijn, A.J.M. Jansman, J.M.J. Rebel, M.A. Smits and
          R.A. Van Emous

17.00h Piglets' peri-weaning intestinal functioning: a multi-suckling system vs
          farrowing crates   66
          S.E. Van Nieuwamerongen, J.E. Bolhuis, C.M.C. Van Der Peet-Schwering, B. Kemp and
          N.M. Soede

Poster Session 03

The effect of chestnut tannins on the prevalence of diarrhea in artificially infected
weaned piglets   67
          S. Thanner, A. Gutzwiller, M. Girard and G. Bee

Effects of the extract of sea buckthorn leaf and berry marc on calves with diarrhoea   68
          L. Liepa, E. Zolnere and I. Dūrītis

Pre-weaning growth affects colonic mucosa response to stress long-after weaning   69
          A. Mereu, J.J. Pastor, C. Dawn, G. Tedo, G. Rimbach and I.R. Ipharraguerre

Development of an *Escherichia coli* challenge model in weaned piglets   70
    X. Guan, M. Van Oostrum, P.J. Van Der Aar and F. Molist

In vitro inhibitory activities of browse extracts on larval exsheathment of goat nematodes 71
    G. Mengistu, H. Hoste, W.H. Hendriks and W.F. Pellikaan

Key issues of poultry gut health and microbiota in Nepal   72
    T. Manoj

Different synbiotic dose feeding effect on the calf digestive channel health and
weight gain   73
    A. Ilgaza and A. Arne

Secondary plant compounds to fight pathogenic and antibiotic resistant bacteria
in farm animals   74
    T. Rothstein and I. Heinzl

Dietary supplementation of quercetin improves performance in weaned piglets   75
    J. Degroote, Z. Ma, H. Vergauwen, W. Wang, N. Van Noten, C. Van Ginneken, S. De Smet
    and J. Michiels

Effects of nutritional interventions on broiler performance, gut microflora and
gene expression   76
    M.M. Van Krimpen, M. Torki and D. Schokker

Antibacterial and immune modulating activities of sulfated polysaccharides of
green algal extract   77
    M. García Suárez, P. Nyvall Collen, F. Bussy, H. Demais and M. Berri

Session 04. Heat stress: consequences and prevention

Chairperson: Dr. David Renaudeau , INRA Rennes
Date: 21 June – 14.00-17.15h
Location: Kleine Veerzaal

Theatre Session 04

14.00h Physiological responses of growing pigs to high ambient temperature
      and/or health challenges   78
  invited *P.H.R.F. Campos, N. Le Floc'h, J. Noblet and D. Renaudeau*

14.45h N-acetyl-L-cysteine improves performance of chronic cyclic heat stressed
      finishing broilers   79
    M. Majdeddin, E. Rosseel, J. Degroote, A. Ovyn, S. De Smet, A. Golian and J. Michiels

15.00h Is rumen temperature a proxy of core body temperature in feedlot cattle? 80
    A.M. Lees, M.L. Sullivan, V. Sejian, J.C. Lees and J.B. Gaughan

15.15h Performance response of grow-finish pigs to a simulated heat stress under
    commercial-like conditions 81
    L.J. Johnston, L.D. Jacobson, B.P. Hetchler, C.D. Reese and A.M. Hilbrands

15.30h Coffee break

16.00h Metabolic profile derangements in heat stressed dairy herds 82
    R.J. Van Saun and J. Davidek

16.15h Early assessment of heat stress-related problem in dairy cows by livestock
    precision farming tools 83
    F. Abeni and A. Galli

16.30h Impact of heat stress on AI and natural service breeding programs in the
    temperate climate 84
    L.K. Schüller and W. Heuwieser

17.00h Effect of heat stress on milk production of Holstein cows in Tunisia 85
    A. Hamrouni and M. Djemali

Poster Session 04

Evaluation of heat stress conditions at cow level inside a dairy barn 86
    L.K. Schüller and W. Heuwieser

Beneficial effect of L-selenomethionine for starter and heat stressed finisher broilers 87
    J. Michiels, J. Degroote, M. Majdeddin, A. Golian, S. De Smet, M. Rovers and L. Segers

Effect of Farm-O-San AHS on performance and blood stress parameters of animals
under heat stress 88
    A. Saiz, J. Mica, S. Chamorro and A.I. García-Ruiz

Heat stress in dairy cows with and without access to shade on pasture in a
temperate climate 89
    E. Van Laer, I. Veissier, R. Palme, C.P.H. Moons, B. Ampe, B. Sonck and F.A.M. Tuyttens

The effect of *Allium sativum* extract on pituitary-gonad axis in heat-stressed female mice 90
    M. Modaresi and M. Heidari

Influence of environmental temperature on the reproductive ability of Holstein cows 91
    S. Doroshchuk, I. Shapiev and E. Nikitkina

Effect of selenium on the growth performance and antioxidant status of stressed
broiler birds 92
B.C. Amaefule, I.E. Uzochukwu and M.C. Ezeokonkwo

Session 05. Adaptation to lactation

Chairperson: Prof. Dr. Helga Sauerwein, University of Bonn
Date: 22 June – 8.30-12.00h
Location: Ir Haakzaal

Theatre Session 05

8.30h Prevention of hypocalcemia in periparturient dairy cows: the key role
       of serotonin   93
       L.E. Hernández-Castellano, L.L. Hernandez, S. Weaver and R.M. Bruckmaier

8.45h A metabolomics approach to characterize metabolic phenotypes in
       periparturient dairy cows   94
       Á. Kenéz, S. Dänicke, M. Von Bergen and K. Huber

9.00h Association of peripartum serum retinol with metabolic, Inflammatory, and
       oxidative stress in cows   95
       T.H. Herdt, B. Norby, J. Gandy and L.M. Sordillo

9.15h Relationship between adiponectin concentration, BCS and insulin response
       in dry dairy cows   96
       J. De Koster, C. Urh, H. Sauerwein and G. Opsomer

9.30h Customising dry period length to improve adaptation to lactation in dairy cows   97
       invited *A.T.M. Van Knegsel, N. Mayasari, J. Chen, R. Van Hoeij, A. Kok and B. Kemp*

10.00h Extended lactation: an option to improve fertility and productivity in high-
       yielding dairy cows   98
       *M. Kaske, G. Niozas, P. Baling, T. Wagner, S. Wiedemann, M. Feldmann, H. Bollwein and
       G. Tsousis*

10.15h Coffee break

10.45h Production diseases 2.0: surplus or lack of nutrients in transition dairy cows?   99
       invited *J.J. Gross and R.M. Bruckmaier*

11.15h Effects of hyperketonemia within the first six weeks of lactation on milk
       production and fertility   100
       J. Ruoff, S. Borchardt, A. Mahrt and W. Heuwieser

11.30h Diurnal differences in milk composition and their influence on *in vitro* growth of *S. aureus* 101
S.W.F. Eisenberg, E.M. Boerhout, L. Ravesloot, A.J.J.M. Daemen, L. Benedictus, V.P.M.G. Rutten and A.P. Koets

11.45h The effect of dry period length and concentrate level on metabolic health in dairy cows 102
R.J. Van Hoeij, J. Dijkstra, R.M. Bruckmaier, J.J. Gross, T.J.G.M. Lam, B. Kemp and A.T.M. Van Knegsel

Poster Session 05

Estimation of heritability and repeatability for milk fever in Costa Rican dairy cattle 103
A. Saborío-Montero, B. Vargas-Leitón, J.J. Romero-Zúñiga and J. Camacho

Relationship between metabolism and natural autoantibodies in dairy cows with different dry period length 104
N. Mayasari, J. Chen, G. De Vries Reilingh, J.J. Gross, R.M. Bruckmaier, B. Kemp, H.K. Parmentier and A.T.M. Van Knegsel

Effects of dry period length on lactation curve characteristics over 2 consecutive years 105
J. Chen, A. Kok, G.J. Remmelink, B. Kemp and A.T.M. Van Knegsel

Alterations of circulating NEFA, BHBA and lipid profile following intravenous glucose administration 106
M. Pourjafar, K. Badiei, A. Chalmeh, M. Mohamadi and F. Momenifar

Performance and long-chain fatty acids in milk and blood of dairy cows fed a corn silage-based diet 107
C. Weber, A. Tröscher, A. Starke, H. Kienberger, M. Rychlik and H.M. Hammon

Adipose tissue INSR and GLUT4 expression with reference to body condition score in Holstein cows 108
H. Jaakson, P. Karis, K. Ling, J. Samarütel, A. Ilves, E. Reimann, P. Pärn, R. Bruckmaier, J. Gross and M. Ots

Season of birth affects 305 d milk and fat yield during first lactation in HF heifers 109
M. Van Eetvelde, M. Pierre, L. Vandaele and G. Opsomer

Impact of 25-hydroxyvitamin D3 combined with an acidifying diet on dairy cows' calcium homeostasis 110
I. Cohrs, M.R. Wilkens, E. Azem, B. Schröder and G. Breves

Effects of cinnamon supplementation on performance and metabolic responses of transition dairy cows 111
H. Vakili, A.R. Alizadeh, A. Ghorbani, R.M. Bruckmaier, H. Sauerwein and H. Sadri

Predicting postpartum disorders with prepartum metabolic markers in dairy cows 112
 S.G.A. Van Der Drift, I.M.G.A. Santman-Berends and G.H.M. Counotte

Changes in the serum BHB concentration before and after parturition in Iranian
dairy cows 113
 M. Sakha

Effects of 25-hydroxycholecalciferol on calcium balance and vitamin D
metabolism in sheep 114
 S. Klinger, G. Breves, B. Schröder and M.R. Wilkens

IGF-1 was not predictive for early post partum ketosis in a field study 115
 V. Jacobs, M. Araujo, R. Tietze and M. Schmicke

Optimization of dry cow management can influence natural antibody (Nab) levels
in dairy cows 116
 S. Carp-Van Dijken, I.M.G.A. Santman-Berends, G. Van Schaik, T.J.G.M. Lam and
 I.E.M. Den Uijl

Experiment-corrected milk fat C18:1 cis-9 concentrations as energy status indicator
in dairy cows 117
 S. Jorjong, A.T.M. Van Knegsel, M. Hostens, F. Lannoo, G. Opsomer and V. Fievez

Colostrum composition assessment by on-farm tools at quarter and composite
level in dairy cows 118
 J.J. Gross, E.C. Kessler and R.M. Bruckmaier

Colostral immunoglobulin concentration is repeatable in consecutive lactations of
dairy cows 119
 J.J. Gross, G. Schüpbach-Regula and R.M. Bruckmaier

Metabolite profiles in blood and milk for cows with different dry period lengths in
early lactation 120
 W. Xu, A.T.M. Van Knegsel, D.B. De Koning, R. Van Hoeij, B. Kemp and J.J.M. Vervoort

Changing patterns of thyroid hormones following bolus intravenous glucose
administration in sheep 121
 K. Badiei, M. Pourjafar, A. Chalmeh, A. Mirzaei, M.H. Zarei and I. Saadat Akhtar

Session 06. Economics of disease

Chairperson: Prof. Dr. Henk Hogeveen, Wageningen UR
Date: 22 June – 13.30-15.15h
Location: Ir Haakzaal

Theatre Session 06

13.30h Comparing the economic impact of production diseases in dairy cattle between countries 122
invited *M. Van Der Voort and H. Hogeveen*

14.15h Economic impact of gastrointestinal parasitic infection on fattening of Desert Sheep 123
N. Eisa, S. Babiker and H. Abdalla

14.30h Impact of different production systems on health care costs in the Dutch broiler farms 124
E. Gocsik, H.E. Kortes, A.G.J.M. Oude Lansink and H.W. Saatkamp

14.45h Economic losses due to subclinical ketosis and related disorders in dairy herds of Iran 125
M. Sakha and S. Nejat Dehkordi

15.00h Economic decision-making on reducing risks of human exposure to AMR through livestock supply chains 126
J.L. Roskam, E. Gocsik, A.G.J.M. Oude Lansink, M.L.W. Schut and H.W. Saatkamp

Poster Session 06

The devastating effects of foot-and-mouth disease in dairy farm 127
A. Hayirli, M. Cengiz, M.O. Timurkan, S. Cengiz, B. Balli and F. Hira

Economic weights for health traits in livestock 128
M. Michaličková, Z. Krupová, E. Krupa and L. Zavadilová

Session 07. Free communications 1

Chairperson: Dr. Gert van Duinkerken, Wageningen UR Livestock Research
Date: 22 June – 14.15-15.30h
Location: Kleine Veerzaal

Theatre Session 07

14.15h Occurrences of production diseases in grower pigs on Irish pig farms 129
N. Van Staaveren, B. Doyle, A. Hanlon and L. Boyle

14.30h Associations between tail lesions and lung health in slaughter pigs 130
  N. Van Staaveren, A. Vale, E.G. Manzanilla, B. Doyle, A. Hanlon and L. Boyle

14.45h Relationship between 'pig flow' from birth to slaughter and the risk of
    disease at slaughter 131
  *J. Calderon-Diaz, L.A. Boyle, A. Diana, F.C. Leonard, M. Mcelroy, S. Mcgettrick,
  J. Moriarty and E.G. Manzanilla*

15.00h A novel scoring system for the classification of the health status of
    growing-finishing pig farms 132
  *A.J.M. Jansman, E. Kampman-Van De Hoek, P. Sakkas, H. Van Beers-Schreurs,
  C.M.C. Van Der Peet-Schwering, J.J.G.C. Van Den Borne and W.J.J. Gerrits*

15.15h Management factors associated with mortality of dairy calves 133
  L. Seppä-Lassila, K. Sarjokari, M. Hovinen, T. Soveri and M. Norring

Poster Session 07

Network for evaluation of One Health: working together for improved health of
the global community 134
  J. Starič, F. Farci and B. Häsler

Epidemiological study of growth performance and carcass quality in pigs fed a
low or high complexity 135
  H. Reinhardt, C.F.M. De Lange and V. Farzan

Induced copper deficiency in a sheep flock 136
  R.J. Van Saun

Effect of restricted feeding on rumen fermentation of Japanese Black fattening
steers during summer 137
  Y. Maeda, K. Nishimura and S. Kushibiki

Evaluation of serum passive transfer status in calves and colostrum with the Brix
refractometer 138
  H. Batmaz and O. Topal

Effects of vitamin and element supplementation on weight gain of calves fed raw
or pasteurised milk 139
  Z. Mecitoglu and H. Batmaz

Session 08. PROHEALTH: Sustainable control of pig and poultry production disease

Chairperson: Prof. Dr. Ilias Kyriazakis, Newcastle University
Date: 23 June – 8.30-12.00h
Location: Ir Haakzaal

Theatre Session 08

8.30h *Escherichia coli* in industrial poultry production: aspects of transmission and disease development 140
invited J.P. Christensen, S.E. Pors, S. Papasolomontos, L.L. Poulsen, I. Thøfner, R.H. Olsen, H. Christensen and M. Bisgaard

9.00h Infections with Gram positive cocci in broiler breeders: significance and prevalence 141
I. Thøfner, L.L. Poulsen, R.H. Olsen, H. Christensen, M. Bisgaard and J.P. Christensen

9.15h Effect of selection for growth rate on the resistance and tolerance of broilers to *Eimeria maxima* 142
P. Sakkas, I. Oikeh, R.A. Bailey, M.J. Nolan, D.P. Blake, A. Oxley, G. Lietz and I. Kyriazakis

9.30h Control of dysbacteriosis in broilers by means of drinking water acidification 143
A. Cools, H. Slagter, C. D Moor, A. Lauwaerts and W. Merckx

9.45h Effect of genetic selection and physical activity on lameness and osteochondrosis prevalence in pigs 144
invited A. Boudon, M. Karhapää, H. Siljander-Rasi, N. Le Floc'h, E. Cantaloube and M.C. Meunier-Salaün

10.15h Coffee break

10.45h Impact of poor hygiene on health and performance of pigs divergently selected for feed efficiency 145
A. Chatelet, E. Merlot, F. Gondret, H. Gilbert and N. Le Floc'h

11.00h Molecular characterisation of idiopathic lumbar kyphosis in pigs 146
A. Clark, I. Kyriazakis, C.R.G. Lewis, R. Farquhar and G. Lietz

11.15h Possible associations between environmental parameters and animal health in two fattening units 147
M. Klinkenberg, L. Vrielinck, D. Demeyer, T. Van Limbergen, E. Lorenzo, G. Montalvo, C. Piñeiro, J. Dewulf and D. Maes

11.30h What are the costs of poultry diseases: a review of nine production diseases 148
P.J. Jones, J. Niemi, R.B. Tranter and R.M. Bennett

11.45h Economic value of mitigating *Actinobacillus pleuropneumoniae* infections in
        pig fattening herds   149
        A.H. Stygar, J.K. Niemi, C. Oliviero, T. Laurila and M. Heinonen

Poster Session 08

Effect of a major gene on piglet response to co-infection with PRRSV and PCV2b   150
        J.R. Dunkelberger, N.V.L. Serao, M. Niederwerder, M.A. Kerrigan, J.K. Lunney,
        R.R.R. Rowland and J.C.M. Dekkers

Reducing ammonia and the risk of disease in agriculture animals   151
        G. Demko, W. Blakeley and P. Pearce

Identification of animal-based traits as indicators of production diseases in pigs   152
        F. Loisel, S. Stravakakis, P. Sakkas, I. Kyriazakis, G. Stewart, N. Le Floc'h and L. Montagne

In vitro cytotoxicity and antiviral activity of plant extracts on avian infectious
bronchitis virus   153
        A. Šalomskas, R. Lelešius, A. Karpovaitė, R. Mickienė, T. Drevinskas, N. Tiso,
        O. Ragažinskienė, L. Kubilienė and A. Maruška

Molecular and functional heterogeneity of the early postnatal satellite cell
population in the pig   154
        K. Stange, C. Miersch, S. Hering, M. Kolisek and M. Röntgen

Antioxidant capacities of pigs were altered in a tissue-specific manner by poor
hygiene conditions   155
        K. Sierzant, E. Merlot, S. Tacher, N. Le Floc'h and F. Gondret

Identifying potential biomarkers to improve production in pigs and poultry   156
        T. Giles, S. Hulme, P. Barrow, N. Le Floc'h, S. Schaeffer, A.M. Chaussé, P. Velge and N. Foster

Session 09. Reproductive disorders in farm animals

Chairperson: Prof. Dr. Matt Lucy, University of Missouri
Date: 23 June – 8.30-12.00h
Location: Kleine Veerzaal

Theatre Session 09

8.30h Interaction between metabolism, immune function and uterine health in
       postpartum dairy cows   157
       invited *G. Opsomer, O. Bogado Pascottini and M. Hostens*

9.15h   Relationships of uterine health with metabolism in dairy cows with
different dry period lengths   158
J. Chen, N.M. Soede, G.J. Remmelink, R.M. Bruckmaier, B. Kemp and A.T.M. Van Knegsel

9.30h   Automatically recorded body condition scores: patterns and associations
with fertility   159
U. Emanuelson, S. Granz and C. Hallén Sandgren

9.45h   Interaction between conception, mastitis and subclinical ketosis in dairy cows   160
A. Albaaj, G. Foucras and D. Raboisson

10.00h Lymphoid aggregates are associated with reduced placental mass and
embryonic loss in dairy cows   161
M.C. Lucy, T.J. Evans and S.E. Poock

10.15h Coffee break

10.45h Hepatic mineral concentrations and health status in bovine fetuses   162
R.J. Van Saun

11.00h Searching for an effective BVD eradication program for the Netherlands   163
D.A. Kalkowska, M. Werkman, A.A. De Koeijer and W.H.M. Van Der Poel

11.15h Relationship between ovulation rate in sows and litter characteristics at birth   164
*C.L.A. Da Silva, D.B. De Koning, B.F.A. Laurenssen, H.A. Mulder, E.F. Knol, B. Kemp and
N.M. Soede*

11.30h Lactational oestrus in group housed lactating sows   165
*B.F.A. Laurenssen, J.E.M. Strous, S.E. Van Nieuwamerongen, J.E. Bolhuis,
C.M.C. Van Der Peet-Schwering and N.M. Soede*

11.45h Influence of fiber and amino acids on farrowing process, sow health and
piglet vitality   166
X. Benthem De Grave, P. Van Der Aar and F. Molist

Poster Session 09

Role of arcuate nucleus-kisspeptin/neurokinin b neurons in control of
reproduction in cows   167
*A.S.A. Hassaneen, M. Kato, Y. Suetomi, Y. Naniwa, T. Sasaki, N. Ieda, N. Inoue, K. Kimura,
S. Oishi, N. Fujii, S. Matsuyama, R. Misu, S. Minabe, H. Tsukamura, F. Matsuda and
S. Ohkura*

The telemetric measurement of the reticulorumen and vaginal acidity and
temperature of dairy cows   168
R. Antanaitis, G. Zamokas, A. Grigonis and V. Žilaitis

Proximal teat amputation in a Brown-Swiss cow with a severe udder oedema 169
P. Steckeler, C. Straub, M. Hipp and W. Petzl

Comparison of two different protocols for induction of parturition in heifers with or without estrad 170
H. Hamali, N. Mehrvar and A. Saberivand

The effects of FSH treatment in Ovsynch protocol on pregnancy rate in dairy cows 171
G. Yilmazbas-Mecitoglu, A. Gumen, A. Keskin, E. Karakaya, U. Tasdemir and A. Alkan

Study on the effect of retained fetal membranes on the reproductive performance in dairy cattle 172
I. Elbawab, M. Elbehiry, M. Marey, K. Metwally and F. Hussein

Session 10. Welfare and production trade-offs

Chairperson: Dr. Bas Rodenburg / Dr. Liesbeth Bolhuis, Wageningen UR
Date: 23 June – 13.30-17.00h
Location: Ir Haakzaal

Theatre Session 10

13.30h Optimising welfare and economic performance in alternative farrowing and lactation systems 173
invited *E.M. Baxter and S.A. Edwards*

14.15h Environmental and social enrichment reduces susceptibility to co-infection in pigs 174
I.D.E. Van Dixhoorn, I. Reimert, J.E. Bolhuis, P.W.G. Groot Koerkamp, B. Kemp and N. Stockhofe-Zurwieden

14.30h Cost-efficiency of animal welfare in broiler prodcution systems 175
E. Gocsik, S.D. Brooshooft, I.C. De Jong and H.W. Saatkamp

14.45h Selection for or against feather pecking: what are the consequences? 176
J.A.J. Van Der Eijk, A. Lammers, B. Kemp, M. Naguib and T.B. Rodenburg

15.00h Coffee break

15.30h Keeping pigs with intact tails: from science to practice 177
M. Kluivers-Poodt, N. Dirx, C.M.C. Van Der Peet, A. Hoofs, W.W. Ursinus, J.E. Bolhuis and G.F.V. Van Der Peet

15.45h Genetic association between early calfhood health status and subsequent performance of dairy cows 178
M. Mahmoud, T. Yin and S. König

16.00h Enrichment materials for intensively-farmed pigs: from review to preview   179
  M.B.M. Bracke

16.15h A survey of straw use and tail biting in Swedish undocked pig farms   180
  T. Wallgren, R. Westin and S. Gunnarsson

16.30h Prevalence of production diseases in organic dairy herds in Germany,
  Spain, France, and Sweden   181
  M. Krieger, A. Madouasse, K. Sjöström, U. Emanuelson, I. Blanco-Penedo, J.E. Duval,
  N. Bareille, C. Fourichon and A. Sundrum

16.45h Effect of hatching conditions on indicators of welfare and health in broiler
  chickens   182
  I.C. De Jong, H. Gunnink, P. De Gouw, F. Leijten, M. Raaijmakers, L. Zoet, E. Wolfs,
  L.F.J. Van De Ven and H. Van Den Brand

Poster Session 10

Bovine practitioner survey: can a new obstetrical instrument really make the difference?   183
  F. Schlederer and A. Wehrend

Dairy cow metabolic status management through productivity and biochemical
compounds of milk   184
  I. Sematovica and L. Liepa

Shoulder ulcers in sows; systemic response and the effect of ketoprofen medication   185
  M. Nystén, T. Orro and O. Peltoniemi

Farm centric and equifinal approach to reduce production diseases on dairy farms   186
  A. Sundrum, U. Emanuelson, C. Fourichon, H. Hogeveen, R. Tranter and A. Velarde

Session 11. Free communications 2

Chairperson: Dr. Gert van Duinkerken, Wageningen UR Livestock Research
Date: 23 June – 15.30-17.00h
Location: Kleine Veerzaal

Theatre Session 11

15.30h Refusal to drink in calves in German farms: phenolic compounds a problem?   187
  M. Höltershinken

15.45h The association between young stock management and antibiotic use in
  young calves   188
  M. Holstege, A. De Bont-Smolenaars, I. Santman-Berends, G. Witteveen, A. Velthuis and
  T. Lam

16.00h Monitoring of antimicrobial use and the association with cattle health
    parameters in the Netherlands   189
    H. Brouwer, I.M.G.A. Santman-Berends, M.A. Gonggrijp, J.J. Hage, A. Smolenaars and
    G. Van Schaik

16.15h The relationship between feed intake and cow behaviour   190
    S. Van Der Beek, R.M. De Mol, R.M.A. Goselink and H.M. Knijn

16.30h A new endoscopic approach for bronchoalveolar lavage at cattle-for better
    results in BRD diagnostics   191
    W. Hasseler and F. Schlederer

16.45h Effects of herd health management on animal health in organic dairy herds
    in Sweden   192
    K. Sjöström and U. Emanuelson

Poster Session 11

Reticular pH as a means of diagnosing subacute ruminal acidosis (SARA) in
periparturient cows   193
    S. Sato, Y. Watanabe, T. Ichijo, M. Maeda and H. Yano

Improvement in the capabilities of a wireless transmission pH measuring system   194
    H. Mizuguchi, N. Kakizaki, K. Ito, D. Kishi and S. Sato

Evaluation of a new portable blood cow side test for calcium   195
    M. Neumayer and H. Hilmert

Connection between biochemical blood indicators of calcium metabolism and BCS   196
    J. Starič, M. Klinkon, M. Nemec and J. Ježek

Evaluation of levels of Ca, free triiodothyronine, free thyroxine and insulin in cows
with ketosis   197
    S. Kozat

Impact of fatty acid supplementation on basal adenosine triphosphate release
from bovine erythrocyte   198
    D. Revskij, S. Haubold, T. Viergutz, C. Weber, A. Tuchscherer, A. Tröscher, H.J. Schuberth,
    H.M. Hammon and M. Mielenz

A new and simple methode to deal with teat injuries   199
    F. Schlederer

Reduced ivermectin efficacy against *Ostertagia* in a Dutch cattle herd   200
    M. Holzhauer, C. Hegeman and D. Van Doorn

Session 12. Burgers Zoo Excursion

Theatre Session 12

Animal health management in Burgers' Zoo   201
    C. Mager

Early lameness detection, cow comfort and infectious lesion control: lessons from the UK

N. Bell
RVC, Production and Population Health, Highwood, Smugglers Lane, Colehill, Wimborne, Dorset,
BH21 2RY, United Kingdom; njbell@rvc.ac.uk

Foot health remains a major priority for improvement in UK dairy systems and worldwide with an estimated 22% of dairy cows lame at any one time in the UK. Rising milk yields, increasing herd size and a growing reliance on unskilled labour will only intensify risk factors. Identifying strategies for improving foot health remains a focus for UK research. One major risk factor is the delay to treatment with many cows lame for over 65 days before receiving treatment, if treated at all. While self-cure appears to be a regular occurrence, delays to treatment in the foot crush may be contributing treatment failures and a creeping rise in lameness levels. Different approaches to reporting lameness are required to understand the dynamics of a multifactorial disease. For example, overall lameness levels for cows with a new case may be as high as 85% 18 weeks after onset, with almost 10% of cows remaining persistently lame. With disciplined scoring approaches and effective treatment it is possible to reduce lameness levels to acceptable levels by today's standards. However, how do we prevent the next wave of lame cows and work to higher standards for the industry in the future. In a series of studies including several randomised control trials we have reported cure rates for lame cows treated early, demonstrated the relevance of deep bedding for achieving optimal lying times, raised concerns over the use of routine foot trimming in large sand units and illustrated the potential benefits of regular foot disinfection protocols for reducing digital dermatitis levels. The conclusions of this work is that through a combination of effective treatment and prevention, producers can potentially achieve high standards of foot health in intensively managed systems.

Gait cycle in dairy cows and its application to detect lameness

M. Alsaaod[1], T. Hausegger[2], R. Kredel[2] and A. Steiner[1]
[1]Clinic for Ruminants, Vetsuisse-Faculty, University of Bern, Bremgartensstrasse 109a, 3012
Bern, Switzerland, [2]Institute of Sport Science, Faculty of Human Sciences, University of Bern,
Bremgartenstrasse 145, 3012 Bern, Switzerland; maher.alsaaod@vetsuisse.unibe.ch

This study evaluated the feasibility of high frequency accelerometers (400 Hz) to measure gait cycle parameters of stance and swing phases in dairy cows. It was hypothesized that an accelerometer with a high sampling rate (400 Hz) allows for: (1) accurate identification and description of the gait cycle pattern in cattle compared to the high speed camera output; and (2) a clear distinction between healthy and affected limbs in lame cows. The experimental study was carried out at the Clinic for Ruminants, Vetsuisse-Faculty, University of Bern, Switzerland. Twelve dairy cows without any visible signs of lameness (C) and five lame cows (L) referred to the clinic were used. The measurements of acceleration were carried out in groups C and L during walking into two sessions: Session (I) assessed the acceleration of the metatarsus (MT) and lateral claw of the same limb simultaneously; session (II) assessed the acceleration of the MT of both hind limbs simultaneously to compare the acceleration between left and right MT and calculate the difference for each variable separately (Δ). The variables of gait cycle included: (1) several amplitudes (preswing, swing, foot load, ratio of preswing to foot load and the ratio of swing to foot load phase); and (2) temporal events (relative duration of stance phase and swing phase to gait cycle and of preswing to stance phase). In session (I), the amplitude of preswing, swing and foot load of the lateral claw was significantly higher as compared to the respective MT ($P<0.05$). The temporal events of the gait cycle, including the relative duration of stance and swing phases of the claw were highly correlated with the MT (rs>0.71), and only the relative duration of the preswing to stance phase was significantly higher at the level of the MT as compared to the claw ($P<0.05$). In session (II), amplitudes and relative temporal events of the gait cycle were not significantly different and moderately to highly correlated (rs: 0.52-0.95) between left and right MT in group C. In lame cows, the foot-load amplitude was significantly lower. Consequently, these cows showed higher ratios of heel-off and toe-off to foot load, lower stance phase, higher swing phase and preswing phase as compared to healthy cows ($P<0.05$). Measuring the gait cycle variables at the level of the MT, using accelerometers with a high sampling rate (400 Hz) is a promising tool to indirectly explore the acceleration of the claw and determine the effect of orthopedic pathologies on the cows' gait.

Use of extended locomotor behavior characteristics for automated identification of lame dairy cows

G. Beer[1], M. Alsaaod[1], A. Starke[2], G. Regula-Schüpbach[3], H. Müller[2], P. Kohler[1] and A. Steiner[1]
[1]University of Bern, Clinic for Ruminants, Länggassstrasse 124, 3012 Berne, Switzerland, [2]University of Leipzig, Clinic for Ruminants and Swine, An den Tierkliniken 11, 04103 Leipzig, Germany, [3]University of Bern, Veterinary Public Health Institute, Schwarzenburgstrasse 155, 3097 Liebefeld, Switzerland; maher.alsaaod@vetsuisse.unibe.ch

This study was carried out firstly to detect differences in locomotor and feeding behavior between lame (group L) and non-lame (group C) cows and secondly to create an automatic lameness detection model, using data of the three-dimensional acceleration of the hind limbs and activity of the jaw. Twelve non-lame and 41 lame multiparous German Holstein cows, housed in a commercial loose stall in Germany, were included in the study. They were equipped with two three dimensional accelerometers (RumiWatch®), attached to each hind limb, and one halter with noseband sensor (RumiWatch®) attached to the head. Accelerometers and noseband sensors had previously been validated. The devices recorded data of 3 consecutive days (recording period). Using video recordings, each cow's gait was scored on a 5-point scale before and after the recording period, and the mean value of 3 independent experienced observers was taken as definite gait score. Group C cows were defined as showing a gait score ≤2, group L as showing a gait score ≥2.5. For comparison between group L and group C, the T-test, the Aspin-Welch test and the Wilcoxon test and for model creation, logistic regression and receiver operating characteristics (ROC) were used. Group L had compared to group C significant lower eating and ruminating time, fewer eating chews, ruminating chews and ruminating boluses, longer lying time and lying bout duration, lower standing time, fewer standing and walking bouts, fewer, slower and shorter strides and a lower walking speed ($P<0.0001$-0.04), whereas ruminating chews per minute and ruminating chews per bolus, as well as walking time and number of lying bouts did not differ between group C and group L ($P>0.09$-0.8). Using only accelerometer variables, we could create a model with a sensitivity and a specificity of >90%. Additional use of noseband sensor data did not substantially improve the model. The results of this study show that the newly developed RumiWatch® accelerometers are able to detect differences in a broad set of behavioral parameters in lame and non-lame cows. Models respecting two accelerometers variables only, automatically identified lame cows with high accuracy. Management factors influence the behavior of dairy cows. Thus, a multicenter study is needed, taking into consideration various management conditions.

Use of routine collected herd data to estimate claw health in dairy herds

H. Brouwer[1], T. Dijkstra[1], H. Worm[1], Y. Van Der Vorst[2] and G. Van Schaik[1]
[1]GD Animal Health, Arnsbergstraat 7, 7418 EZ Deventer, the Netherlands, [2]Royal Friesland Campina, Stationsplein 4, 3818 LE Amersfoort, the Netherlands; h.brouwer@gdanimalhealth.com

Lameness in dairy cattle is a serious welfare issue, it is highly prevalent and associated with high treatment costs. Claw health is one of the three focus points (besides udder health and fertility) that need to be improved in order to enhance a sustainable dairy production. The claw health status of a herd can be assessed by clinical observation of individual cows, which is time consuming and may be associated with a large variability between observers. The objective of the study was to develop an empirical model on routine collected herd data that could classify herds with a below or above average claw health. Two hundred dairy herds were visited by a trained veterinarian to determine the percentage of lame cows, the percentage of cows with visible hock or knee lesions and an overall grade for claw health. Routine collected herd data were obtained and converted into cattle health parameters, concerning fertility, milk quality, mortality and herd health data. Principal component analysis was used to combine the claw health parameters from the herd visit into a continuous observed claw health score. Herds were classified as below (score<0) or above average (score≥0) for claw health. The dataset was randomly divided in a test group of 150 herds to develop a predictive model and a group of 50 herds for validation of the model. Multivariable linear regression with a backward elimination procedure was carried out on routine herd data of the test group to find the best predictive model for claw health. With the final predictive model, the claw health status of the 50 validation herds was estimated. The agreement between the predicted relative to the observed claw health score was obtained and the sensitivity and specificity of the model were determined using the veterinary observations as gold standard. The final predictive model explained 27% of the variance in the observed claw health score and contained cattle mortality, non-ear tagged calf mortality, replacement rate, no. of inseminations per cow, purchase of cattle in the last year and the herd status for bovine viral diarrhea, *Salmonella* and infectious bovine rhinotracheitis. The model correctly classified the claw health status for 72% of the validation herds with a sensitivity of 77% (95% CI 46-95%) and specificity of 76% (95% CI 57-90%). The study showed that there is merit in estimating claw health of dairy farms using routine collected herd data. This provides the opportunity to monitor claw health in a population. The claw health status of individual herds combined with a benchmark may stimulate herd owners to improve claw health in their herds.

Digital dermatitis in dairy cattle: infectivity of the different stages

F. Biemans[1,2], P. Bijma[1] and M.C.M. De Jong[2]
[1]*Wageningen UR, Animal Breeding and Genomics Centre, P.O. Box 338, 6700 AH Wageningen, the Netherlands,* [2]*Wageningen UR, Quanitative Veterinary Epidemiology, P.O. Box 338, 6700 AH Wageningen, the Netherlands; floor.biemans@wur.nl*

Digital Dermatitis (DD) is an infectious claw disease of cattle caused by bacteria, mainly Treponemes, that is transmitted between animals. The disease causes ulcerative lesions usually occurring along the coronary band of the hind claws. DD is associated with lameness, which has a negative effect on the welfare of animals and causes economic losses. DD lesions can be classified into six distinct stages (M0-M4.1), each with their own characteristics: M0 is the healthy stage, M1 is the early stage of DD with a lesion of 0-2 cm in diameter, M2 indicates classical ulceration of DD with a lesion diameter >2 cm, M3 lesions are covered by a scab, M4 is the chronic stage with a dyskeratotic lesion, and stage M4.1 is a small lesion (M1) in addition to a chronic infection (M4). Still little is known about the progression and transmission of DD. It is straightforward that the M0 stage, where DD lesions are absent, is classified as susceptible. The remaining stages are classified as infected based on clinical appearance. The total infectiousness of a stage is the product of the transmission rate per day and the duration of the stage. Together, the (infectious) stages determine the basic reproduction ratio (R_0). R_0 indicates how many infections are on average caused by a typically infected individual. The aim of this study was to estimate R_0 and the contribution of each stage to this number. Data were collected on twelve farms in the Netherlands. Every two weeks, for half a year, both hind claws of all milked cows were scored for DD lesion stage. The transmission rate per day for the different stages was estimated using a Generalized Linear Model with a log-log link function. Next, the average sojourn time was calculated for each infected stage. Differences in transmission rate per day between stages were small, with transmission rates per day of 0.026, 0.014, 0.049, 0.031 and 0.0084 for stage M1, M2, M3, M4 and M4.1, respectively. Only the transmission rates for stage M2 and M3 differed significantly. 92.5% of the DD infections was first observed as a chronic lesion (M4), other lesions became relatively soon an M4 lesion as well. Moreover, the sojourn time in the M4 stage was very long compared to the other stages. The basic reproduction ratio (R_0) was 2.2. So, differences in transmission rate were small and infected animals had an M4 lesion the majority of the time. Therefore, M4 lesions are the most important and determine R_0. Thus, the focus should be on this lesion stage when measures are taken to lower the prevalence of DD.

Prevalence, risk factors and bacterial species associated with non-healing white line disorders

E. Van Engelen, M. Gonggrijp, M. Holzhauer, A. Ten Wolthuis and A. Velthuis
GD Animal health, P.O. Box 9, 7400 AA Deventer, the Netherlands; e.v.engelen@gddiergezondheid.nl

Lameness is an important cause of reduced welfare in dairy cow herds in the Netherlands. Additionally, lameness increases the risk of cows to be culled early. Since one decade, dairy farmers are confronted by a new claw disorder causing chronic severe lameness, described as non-healing white line disorder (NHWLD). In this study the prevalence, risk factors and etiology of NHWLD on animal and farm level were studied. To gain insight in the prevalence,185 farms were visited and digital claw health recordings in the period 2011-2012 were analyzed. Additionally, 140 farmers completed a survey with regard to potential risk factors. To determine if and which bacteria may contribute to NHWLD, from three farms six claw horn samples from claws with NHWLD and six from claws with regular lesions (e.g. sole ulcer, white line lesion) were analyzed. The samples were cultured both under aerobic and anaerobic conditions on selective media and bacteria were identified with MALDI-TOF MS. Bacteria that couldn't be identified with MALDI-TOF were clustered with MALDI-TOF software. From 45 clusters, 4 had a relationship with NHWLD. The bacteria belonging to these clusters were identified using 16S rDNA sequencing. Finally, presence of *Dichelobacter nodosus* was determined with PCR. In 2011, NHWLD was diagnosed on 72% (95% ci: 64-78%) of the farms. In 2012 this was 76% (95% ci: 69-82%). The median prevalence on animal level was 3% (range: 0-24%) in 2011. In 2012 this was 4% (range: 0-20%). At animal level NHWLD was associated with interdigital dermatitis and negatively associated with digital dermatitis. On farm level NHWLD was associated with the hoof trimming organization, a previous BVD infection and negatively associated with different grazing schemes, hoof trimming schedule and hygiene practices. 29 different bacterium species could be identified. Clusters that were associated with NHWLD belonged to the genus *Prevotella* or *Porphyromonas*. Other bacteria that might be associated with NHWLD were *Fusobacterium* and *Bacteroides* and *Dichelobacter nododus*. We conclude that certain strict anaerobic bacteria like *Prevotella*, *Bacteroides*, *Fusobacterium* and *Dichelobacter nodosus* were associated with a common cause of chronic lameness in dairy cattle, described as non-healing white line disorder. Additionally we could describe three risk factors for this disorder both on animal and farm level, and four protective factors.

Perceptions about the causes, treatment and prevention of lameness in a pasture-based dairy industry

J. Marchewka[1,2], J.F. Mee[2] and L.A. Boyle[2]
[1]Institute of Genetics and Animal Breeding of the Polish Academy of Sciences, Department of Animal Behaviour, ul. Postepu 36A, Jastrzębiec, 05-552 Magdalenka, 05-552 Magdalenka, Poland, [2]Teagasc, Animal and Grassland Research and Innovation Centre, Moorepark, Fermoy, Co. Cork, NA, Ireland; joanna.marchewka@teagasc.ie

Lameness is an important welfare problem for dairy cows irrespective of the production system. The key preventive measures for the control of lameness include good infrastructure, foot-bathing and hoof paring. This study aimed to investigate the perceptions of key stakeholders about lameness in Irish dairy cows. The survey was conducted with dairy farmers (F; n=115) at two national farming events (National Ploughing Championships and Moorepark Open Day 2015) and cattle veterinarians (V; n=60) at the Cattle Association of Veterinary Ireland conference by interview. Teagasc dairy advisors were asked to complete the survey themselves (A; n=48) at an 'in-service' training day. The 223 respondents were asked to: identify the 1° type of lameness (L) in Irish dairy cows and how best to treat and prevent it. The results are expressed as a % of each group surveyed. A Chi-Square Fisher test was used to investigate differences in distributions of response frequencies between groups using PROC FREQ in SAS. Stakeholders agreed (χ^2=3.0; P=0.2224) that the most common causes of L in Irish pasture based systems are likely to be white line disease (WLD) and digital dermatitis (DD). Stakeholders did not differ in their opinions about the best way of preventing WLD (χ^2=22; P=0.078) with the majority in all stakeholders groups indicating the importance of good roadways (A: 42.86%; F: 55.56%; V: 35.71%). However, stakeholders disagreed on the best way of preventing DD (χ^2=32.9091; P<0.0001). A differed strongly from F on the importance of 'hoof care' (0 vs 70.37%) and 'good roadways' (30.77 vs 0%). There were also knowledge gaps and disagreement between A and F, as to whether the best way to treat WLD (χ^2=9.6; P=0.0082) is footbathing (42.86% and 8.33% respectively) or paring (57.14% and 91.67% respectively). F responses did not differ from V. There was also disagreement on the best way of treating DD (χ^2=22; P=0.0373). A significantly lower proportion of A (38.5%) selected footbathing as the 1° treatment for DD compared to F (66.7%) with V being intermediary (42.9%). Encouragingly knowledge levels of basic lameness issues were good amongst farmers and in certain cases did not differ from vets. However the importance of management and a housing environment that maximises cow comfort cannot be underestimated in lameness prevention. Given the importance of the role of advisory services in transferring knowledge on such issues there appears to be a need for further education of dairy advisors about lameness prevention and treatment.

The effect of rubber-covered floors on gait and claw lesions in group-housed gestating sows

E.-J. Bos[1,2], D. Maes[1], M. Van Riet[1,2], S. Millet[1,2], B. Ampe[2], G. Janssens[1] and F. Tuyttens[1,2]
[1]Ghent University, Faculty of Veterinary Medicine, Salisburylaan 133, 9820 Merelbeke, Belgium, [2]Institute for Agricultural and Fisheries Research, Animal Science Unit, Scheldeweg 68, 9090 Melle, Belgium; emiliejulie.bos@ilvo.vlaanderen.be

Lameness and claw lesions in sows are major welfare and production problems. The prevalence of these problems has been reported to be higher in group housing systems with hard flooring, such as concrete floors. In a 2x3 factorial design, we investigated the effect of rubber top layers on concrete floors and the effect of three levels of zinc supplementation in the feed on gait and claw lesions in group-housed sows. Six groups of 21±4 hybrid sows were monitored during three successive reproductive cycles. The sows were group-housed from d28 after insemination (d0) until one week before expected farrowing date (d108) in pens with either concrete floors or concrete floors covered with rubber in part of the lying area and in the full slatted area. During each reproductive cycle, gait was assessed four times (d28, d50, d108 and d140), and claw lesions were assessed twice (d50 and d140). The data were analysed using a linear mixed model with floor, feed, phase in cycle and their interactions as fixed effects and parity, group and sow as random effects. Here we report on the effect of floor type, which did not interact with dietary zinc concentration ($P>0.10$ for all outcome variables). Gait and claw scores are given in mm, on visual analogue scales of 150 and 160 mm, respectively. Results are given as means ± SD. Gait scores of sows housed on rubber flooring at d108 were better than for sows housed on concrete flooring (43±27 vs 53±31 mm; $P<0.001$). Mean lameness prevalence was higher ($P<0.05$) during the group-housing phase (d28-d108; 26.4%) as compared to individual-housing phases (d108-d28 of the next cycle; 6.6%). But, no differences in lameness prevalence were found between floor types, irrespective of the phase in the reproductive cycle ($P=0.341$). Regarding claw disorders, at mid-group (d50) rubber-covered floors scored 4.6±1.8 mm better for 'heel overgrowth and erosion' ($P=0.01$) and 3.1±1.5 mm for 'heel–sole crack' ($P=0.04$). However, rubber-covered floors scored 3.4±1.7 mm worse for 'vertical cracks in the wall horn' ($P=0.04$) at d50. At the end of lactation (d140) rubber-covered floors scored 2.9±1 mm better for 'white line' ($P=0.02$) and 4.7±1.4 mm for 'claw length' ($P<0.001$). Claw lesion prevalence at d50 was lower compared to d140 (84.6 vs 94.8%; $P<0.001$), but there was no floor effect. The improved scores for gait and some claw characteristics towards the end of gestation suggest that rubber-topped floors in the group housing unit have a beneficial effect on the gait and claw lesions of sows.

Physical exercise of dairy cows: effects of training on activity, lying behaviour and heart rate

W. Ouweltjes, G.P. Binnendijk and R.M.A. Goselink
Wageningen UR, Livestock Research, De Elst 1, 6708 WD Wageningen, the Netherlands;
wijbrand.ouweltjes@wur.nl

Dairy cows housed in cubicle barns generally have very limited physical activity, because all resources they need are nearby. This is a clear distinction with the situation under natural circumstances or for grazing cattle. For humans remarkable positive effects are known of physical activity both on physical and mental health. Therefore it is hypothesised that increased exercise of housed dairy cows stimulates their fitness and that this in turn can increase health and longevity. Thus it also could contribute to one of the ambitions of the Dutch dairy industry. An experiment was conducted where 18 lactating cows received 45 minutes of training twice daily (Monday-Friday) in a treadmill (STEP group) after morning milkings and before afternoon milkings and 18 control cows (CON group) did not. Apart from the training they were kept under similar circumstances and fed the same diets for an experimental period of 8 weeks. The animals were milked twice daily in a conventional parlour. Activity of all animals was monitored with IceQubes® throughout the experiment (measurements started in the week preceding the experiment), heart rates were measured once weekly for 3 indicator cows per group starting after the morning exercise and ending after the afternoon milking with Zephyr Bioharness™ sensors. In the post experimental week all animals were habituated to wearing a belt around the chest and walk around in the treadmill for a while. After 3 days of habituation all cows were walked around in the treadmill for 10 minutes with Bioharness™ sensors mounted around their chest. These sensors were removed and stopped around 15 minutes after the animals were back in the barn. Results indicate that the STEP group had significantly more steps throughout the experimental period than the CON group (2,612 vs 949 per cow per day), so the training indeed did increase their overall activity, but only during days when they were trained. Differences between individual animals were substantial. However, training did not significantly affect overall time budgets for lying and standing or bout lengths, although the STEP cows on average lay down significantly more in the weekends than the CON cows (58.3 vs 51.2% of time), but this was already the case before training started. Preliminary investigations show that heart rates substantially increased during training, indicating the effort of the training was considerable. The impact of training on recovery after a physical challenge is currently under investigation. Moreover, heart rates while the animals are not challenged will be compared for the two groups.

Physical exercise of dairy cows: effects of training on energy balance
R.M.A. Goselink, G.P. Binnendijk and W. Ouweltjes
Wageningen UR Livestock Research, P.O. Box 338, 6700 AH Wageningen, the Netherlands;
roselinde.goselink@wur.nl

Dairy cows housed indoors are physically less active than cows under grazing conditions. The level of physical activity of cows may however have implications for general health and performance, as shown in other species. The comparison between grazing and indoor housing however is difficult, as other aspects may interfere with the results such as differences in diet (grazing vs indoor), bedding (cubicle vs soil) and hygiene. In this experiment we studied the single effect of a fixed amount of physical exercise of indoor-housed dairy cows on feed intake, milk production and blood parameters relevant for energy metabolism. A group of 36 multiparous lactating Holstein Friesian dairy cows (70-270 DIM) were blocked according to DIM, milk yield and body weight and assigned to one of two treatment groups. Cows in group CON were housed indoors, milked twice daily receiving a diet of 6.7 MJ/d supplemented with 8.7 kg compound concentrate to match energy and nutrient requirements. Cows in group STEP were housed and managed the same, but received additional physical exercise in a treadmill. This training was performed during 8 weeks (wk 1-8) on weekdays by walking 45 minutes at a speed of 3.4 km/h twice daily (5 km/d). Cows were weighed daily, milk composition was analysed weekly and blood samples have been taken in wk 0, 1, 2, 4, 6, 8. Week averages were analysed by REML analysis with treatment and week as fixed factors and cow as random factor. Live weight decreased by 20 kg (-3%) after starting the training in the STEP group and this difference was persistent throughout the trial ($P<0.001$). Dry matter intake tended to decrease for STEP cows in the first 3 weeks of the trial and then returned to the same level as CON cows ($P=0.07$). Milk yield tended to be more persistent in the STEP group ($P=0.09$). Milk fat content increased after starting the training (wk 1 and 2) and returned to CON levels afterwards ($P<0.001$), in parallel with serum NEFA which increased in wk 1 and 2 for STEP cows ($P<0.001$) without affecting BHBA concentration. The training resulted in an increased level of serum creatinine ($P<0.001$) and decreased plasma glucose concentration ($P<0.001$) in the STEP group. In conclusion, increasing dairy cow activity by daily forced physical exercise resulted in higher muscular activity as expected, shown by increased creatinine levels. Due to the exercise, the energy metabolism shifted after a short period of fat mobilisation (high NEFA and milk fat) to a new equilibrium at a decreased plasma glucose concentration. Milk production tended to be more persistent, suggesting that the energy lost to the additional physical exercise does not result in reduced milk production but may improve dairy cow energy metabolism.

Case report: leg lameness in gilts

E. De Jong[1] and P. Bonny[2]
[1]Dierengezondheidszorg Vlaanderen, Deinse Horsweg 1, 9031 Drongen, Belgium,
[2]Praktijkdierenarts, Beselarestraat 187, 8980 Zonnebeke, Belgium; ellen.dejong@dgz.be

In two Belgian farrow-to-finish herds problems of leg weakness occurred in gilts. Danish gilts arrived in Belgium at 20 kg, stayed in quarantine in a rearing unit and were transported to herd 1 at 180-240 days of age. They were fed a rearing diet ad lib. Between eight and ten days after arrival at the herd almost half of the gilts started limping. Only the hind limbs were affected, with discrete swelling of the joints. Gilts purchased from different breeding units in Denmark were directly transported to herd 2, where they were kept in quarantine during 15 weeks. The animals were fed a rearing diet twice a day. Gilts were supplemented with 50g monocalciumphosphate on a weekly basis until farrowing. More than 80% of the gilts showed swelling of the joints, with variable degrees of lameness, starting from one week after arrival. The differential diagnosis of leg weakness in gilts embraces trauma, OCD, deficits in Ca en bacterial infections. Deficits in Ca can be caused by nutritional imbalance. The gilts' quarantine diets were analysed and serological analyses were done of the gilts. Necropsies were performed on two gilts, together with histological and bacteriological examination. No remarkable deficits were discovered in the diets. Serological analyses showed a normal serological Ca concentration. However, concentration of P was too high. Ca/P ratios of >4 have been found. Concentrations of osteocalcin were too low (<11 µg/l), indicative for bad bone turnover or insufficient bone formation. In addition, CTx, a marker of bone mobilization, was too low. Necropsies demonstrated discrete injuries at the cartilage at the femur heads. Both knee joints were filled with hemorrhagic fluid and mild cartilage injuries were present on the condyles. Histological examination revealed distinct hyperplasia and hypertrophia of the synoviae and perivascular infiltration of round cells, being an image of subacute infectious arthritis. Bacteriological examination showed a positive PCR for M. hyosynoviae. The purchased gilts were probably carriers of M. hyosynoviae. During transport to the herds, they were exposed to stress. This caused a penetration of the bacteria in the blood stream, moving to the joints, resulting in discrete arthritis, swelling of the joints and pain, which resulted in limping gilts one to two weeks after arrival. Treatment with high dose antibiotics (macrolides and spectinomycines) and NSAIDs solved the acute problem. To avoid similar problems in the future, preventive measures mainly emphasise avoiding stress (stocking density, housing conditions, transport, etc.). Besides, precaution needs to be taken considering nutritional imbalance and (viral) co-infections.

Effect of hydroxy-copper and -zinc and L-selenomethionine on claw health of sows

A.B.J. Van Dalen and I. Eising

Orffa, Vierlinghstraat 51, 4251 LC Werkendam, the Netherlands; eising@orffa.com

From literature it is known that trace minerals (TM) copper (Cu) and zinc (Zn) influence claw health positively. Selenium (Se) is known to play an important role in inflammation and immunity. On a practical farm with claw health problems, currently used TM $CuSO_4$, $ZnSO_4$ in combination with Zn-chelate and Se-yeast were replaced by hydroxy-Cu and -Zn and L-selenomethionine (L-SeMet). The effect of these higher bioavailable sources on claw health over time was investigated. In the gestation diet 14 ppm $CuSO_4$, 70 ppm $ZnSO_4$ + 37 ppm Zn-chelate and 0.2 ppm Se-yeast were replaced by 14 ppm hydroxy-Cu, 75 ppm hydroxy-Zn and 0.2 ppm L-SeMet. In the lactation diet 16 ppm $CuSO_4$, 80 ppm $ZnSO_4$ + 43 ppm Zn-chelate and 0.2 ppm Se-yeast were replaced by 16 ppm hydroxy-Cu, 85 ppm hydroxy-Zn and 0.2 ppm L-SeMet. A practical farm with 750 sows was used for the trial. Claws of sows in the farrowing room were scored monthly. The claws were scored on five different parameters: cracks and overgrowth of heel area, toe length of by-claw, toe length of inner and outer claw, cracks in horn wall and skin damages above claw. Scores 1-4 were given, 1 being good/healthy, 4 being extremely deviating. The claw score method used was developed by ©Verantwoorde Veehouderij – Wageningen UR (2006). Scores from 1 month before start and of start of the trial were averaged (control) and compared to average scores of 7, 8 and 9 months after TM replacement (treatment). Differences were observed between control and treatment for the amount of severe claw problems (scores 3 and 4). The amount of sows with score 3 and 4 for cracks and overgrowth of the heel area in the control period was 4.32 vs 0.19% in treatment period. The amount of sows with score 3 and 4 for toe length of by-claw in the control period was 0.61 vs 1.37% in the treatment period. Inner and outer claw toe length score 3 and 4 were 1.79% in the control period vs 1.77% in the treatment period. In the control period, 4.88% of the sows had score 3 and 4 for cracks in horn wall compared to 0.78% in treatment period. Score 3 and 4 for skin damages above claw was 10.65% in control period vs 1.35% of the sows in the treatment period. From this trial it was concluded that trace elements have an effect on claw health. Replacing Cu, Zn and Se by the examined better available sources might be a nutritional tool to improve claw health problems in practical situations.

Mycoplasma arthritis outbreaks in dairy herds

M. Holzhauer, R. Dijkman, E. Van Engelen, M.A. Gonggrijp and K. Junker
GD Deventer, P.O. Box 9, 7400 AA Deventer, the Netherlands; m.holzhauer@gddiergezondheid.nl

Mycoplasma outbreaks occurred last 3 years over 50 times in the Netherlands, causing mainly serious painful arthritis in the carpal and fetlock joints of the front leg. In most cases it started suddenly and after 2 months >90% of the cases could be closed as there were no new patients. Herds were initially suspected of mycoplasma infection because of the severity of clinical signs. The average percentage of affected cows within the investigated herds was 7.7% (SD: 4.5%). In 60% of the herds, both arthritis and mastitis problems associated with *Mycoplasma bovis* were observed. In 2 of these herds the same *M. bovis* strain was isolated from the affected joint and the mastitis milk. Respiratory problems of replacement calves were reported in <50 of the herds, while none of the herds showed respiratory problems in the dairy cows. At post mortem examination, affected dairy cows demonstrated acute or chronic serofibrinous to purulent inflammation (septic arthritis) of the frontleg fetlock or carpal joint or the hock joint. One cow suffered from polyarthritis. In addition chronic peri-articular inflammation of the soft tissue (periarthritis) and chronic (necrotizing) mastitis were observed. Consistent with the clinical results no lung lesions were found in any of the examined cows. For welfare reasons, affected cows were culled or euthanized in most herds. A survey was conducted and showed no relationships between clinical disease and parity, stage of lactation or breed. The mean herd size in affected herds was larger (183 dairy cows) than the average herd size in the Netherlands (91 dairy cows; CBS 2013) and herds were mainly located in a certain region of the country. Based on a matched case-control multivariable analysis, case herds were significantly associated with purchase of cattle and a higher protein percentage in milk. All *M. bovis* isolates (from joint infections dairy cows/calves, pneumonia cases calves, and (clinical) mastitis samples) were genotyped using Multi Locus VNTR Analysis (MLVA) typing to determine relatedness of the isolated *M. bovis* isolates both within and between herds and several distinct groups of *M. bovis* isolates could be distinguished. *M. bovis* isolated from affected joints in dairy cows did not form a distinct group as compared to the *M. bovis* isolates from infected lungs in calves, from mastitis and historical samples. Most affected herds were infected by a dominant strain of *M. bovis*, although, in a few herds, different strains of *M. bovis* were isolated from the same herd. There was very little overlap in strains between herds, most herds were associated with herd-specific unique strains. Typing results indicated that the recent outbreaks of *M. bovis* in the Netherlands were not due to entrance or spread of one specific strain rather than due to spread of the species.

Quantification of extended characteristics of locomotor behavior in dairy cows

M. Alsaaod[1], J. Niederhauser[2], G. Schüpbach-Regula[3], G. Beer[1] and A. Steiner[1]
[1]Clinic for ruminants, Vetsuisse-Faculty, University of Bern, Bremgartensstrasse 109a, 3012 Bern, Switzerland, [2]InnoClever GmbH, Tiergartenstrasse 9, 4410 Liestal, Switzerland, [3]Veterinary Public Health Institute, Vetsuisse-Faculty, University of Bern, Schwarzenburgstrasse 155, 3097 Liebefeld, Switzerland; maher.alsaaod@vetsuisse.unibe.ch

Change of animal behavior is one of the most important indicators for assessing cattle health and well-being. Parameters of animal behavior can be used to build up an early disease warning system. The objective of this study was to develop and validate a novel algorithm to monitor locomotor behavior of loose-housed dairy cows based on the output of the RumiWatch® pedometer. It was hypothesized that a novel algorithm of the RumiWatch® pedometer device can be developed that provides a high correlation of parameters of behaviour of dairy cows in both upright and lying positions between the output data of the pedometers and the data derived from temporarily staggered video analysis. Materials and Data of locomotion were acquired by simultaneous pedometer measurements at a sampling rate of 10 Hz and video-recordings for manual observation later. The study consisted of 3 independent experiments. Experiment I was carried out to develop and validate the algorithm for lying behavior, experiment II for walking and standing behavior and experiment III for stride duration and stride length. The final version was validated, using the raw data, collected from cows not included in the development of the algorithm. Spearman correlation coefficients (r_s) were calculated between accelerometer variables and respective data derived from the video recordings (gold standard). Dichotomous data were expressed as the proportion of correctly detected events, and the overall difference for continuous data was expressed as the relative measurement error (RME). In all experiments, the mean difference between accelerometer data and respective gold standard was between 0 and 17% (depending on the variable of locomotion), and the correlation between respective data ranged from r_s=1 to r_s=0.75. The strong to very high correlations of the variables between visual observation and converted pedometer data indicate that the novel RumiWatch® algorithm may markedly improve automated livestock management systems for efficient health monitoring of dairy cows. This study was generously supported by grants of the Fondation Sur-La-Croix (Basel, Switzerland) and the Swiss Federal Commission for Technology and Innovation CTI (Bern, Switzerland) (grant No. 15234.2 PFLS-LS). We thank ITIN+HOCH GmbH, Liestal, Switzerland, for providing the RumiWatch® pedometers for this project.

Effectiveness of copper sulfate solutions in footbaths

A. Prastiwi, Z. Okumus, A. Hayirli, D. Celebi, L. Yanmaz, E. Dogan and U. Ersoz
Ataturk University, Veterinary Medicine, Ataturk University, Erzurum, 25240, Turkey, Turkey;
artinaprastiwi@yahoo.com

Copper sulfate is commonly used antiseptic in dairy farms to prevent hoof diseases. The objectives of this study were to determine the changes in pH of footbath containing copper sulfate ($CuSO_4$) and the types of bacteria in footbath as cow passed. The experiment was conducted in a dairy farm with 360 Holstein and Simmental cows that were milked three times daily in 2×12 herringbone milking parlor. After passing each of 24 cows (passage n=15) from footbath ($220\times90\times15$ cm) containing 0, 2, and 4% $CuSO_4$, the sample was collected from footbath for pH and microbiology. Each treatment was renewed at each milking and tested for 3 days. The loss of antiseptic effectiveness was considered when pH exceeds 5. After determining pH, samples were incubated for 24-72 h for bacterial and fungal growth. Data were analyzed by one-way ANOVA with repeated measures option. The initial and final pH were 7.322-8.240, 4.507-5.198, and 3.643-4.357 for 0, 2, and 4% copper sulfate solution. pH became greater than 5.0 after 7th passage when $CuSO_4$ concentration was 2% and did not exceed 5 even after 15th passage when CuSO4 was 4%. As pH increased after each pH, footbath solution turned from blue to brown. *E. coli* was present at all copper sulfate concentrations, whereas fungus was not present. In conclusion, footbath solution should be monitored for color and changed before it gets alkaline depending upon the number of cow passing for effective hoof disease prevention protocol.

The quality of light and its intensity in housing of poultry: potential effects on behavior

R. Korbel

Clinic for Birds, Reptiles, Amphibians and Ornamental Fish, University Ludwig-Maximilian Munich, Sonnenstrasse 18, 85764 Oberschleissheim/Germany; korbel@vogelklinik.vetmed.uni-muenchen.de

In many bird species – as well as commercially kept poultry species – the eye is the most important sensory organ. The capacities of the avian eye are an adaptation to the specific way of life and habitats as well as physical activities that are closely bound to perfectly functioning vision (e.g. flying). These capacities include: (1) superior visual acuity is mostly exceeding capacities of the human eye; (2) pentrachromatic vision: orientation within five colour channels versus three in man; (3) ultraviolet perception: visual spectrum 320-680 nm; (4) increased flicker fusion frequency. From a practical point of view while keeping birds under artificial light sources two features are of major importance: UV perception and increased flicker fusion frequency. Flicker fusion frequency is the ability of the eye to detect single frames within a certain movement. In the human eye flicker fusion frequency is 16 to 80 frames per seconds (f/s), whereas electroretinograpical (EEG) – studies proof the flicker fusion frequency in many birds to be as high as 160 f/s. A wide variety of specific capacities is closely bound to these visual capacities: (1) intra- and interspecific communication and sexual dimorphism; even in those appearing monomorphic for the human eye, birds are able to differ between males and females by detecting sex-related differences in the UV-reflection of feathers and cutaneous areas; (2) crypsis; insects using camouflage (green insect on a green leaf) can be detected by the avian eye perceiving within the UV; (3) rearing; in various bird species, such as zebra finches, the beak includes highly UV-reflective areas within the beak cavity, used as an optical signal for feeding; (4) assessment of food; Various fruits differ in the ability to reflect within the UV depending on the status of ripeness. Birds assess food using this principle; (5) detection of prey patches; various raptor species (e.g. common kestrels) find prey patches detecting the UV-reflection of urine - an intense UV-reflection is indicative for a dense mouse population. It has to be stressed, that conventional light sources are designed for human vision, not meeting the requirements of the avian eye. Thus keeping pet birds and poultry under artificial light conditions and meeting animal welfare aspects requires light sources emitting within the UV-spectrum (320-380 nm) using so-called 'full spectrum' or 'true light' light sources, at the same time emitting flicker free light, to be realized using a so-called electronic control gear (ECG) or dimmer converting alternate current (AC) to decent current (DC).

New approaches in housing and management to improve foot pad health in fattening poultry

I.C. De Jong and J. Van Harn
Wageningen UR Livestock Research, Animal Welfare, P.O. Box 338, 6700 AH Wageningen, the Netherlands; ingrid.dejong@wur.nl

Footpad dermatitis, a condition of inflammation and necrotic lesions of the plantar surface of the foot, is a common problem in broiler and turkey production, despite the fact that monitoring footpad health has become part of broiler welfare legislation in some European countries. Severe footpad lesions are painful and not only have a negative effect on broiler welfare in itself, but are also related to impaired product quality, impaired technical performance and other welfare problems such as impaired locomotion and increased incidence of hock burns. In Denmark and Sweden, where footpad dermatitis has been monitored already for years, the prevalence in broiler flocks is generally low. However, in other countries there can be a large variation in the prevalence of footpad dermatitis between individual broiler and turkey flocks. Wet and/or sticky litter is generally considered to be the most important causal factor of footpad dermatitis, but there are many housing and management aspects that affect litter quality. In this presentation we will provide an overview of recent studies on management and housing factors influencing litter quality and thus the prevalence of footpad dermatitis in broilers and turkeys, such as feed composition and feed form, bedding type and depth, temperature and relative humidity, drinking water management, light intensity and light programmes. Apart from these factors, (infectious) diseases causing diarrhoea affect the litter quality, and genetic background of the birds also plays a role in the risk to develop footpad dermatitis. More recent studies showed that not only housing or management, but also broiler breeder feeding programmes and incubation conditions may play a role in the risk to develop footpad dermatitis in broiler chickens by affecting the development of the skin of the feet. This area needs further study, because if these relationships indeed exist a production chain approach will help to reduce the incidence of footpad dermatitis in fattening poultry.

Feather pecking and cannibalism in 107 organic laying hen flocks in 8 European countries

M. Bestman[1], C. Verwer[1], F. Smajlhodzic[2], J.L.T. Heerkens[3], L.K. Hinrichsen[4], C. Brenninkmeyer[5], V. Ferrante[6], A. Willet[7] and S. Gunnarsson[8]
[1]Louis Bolk Institute, Hoofdstraat 24, 3972 LA, the Netherlands, [2]University of Veterinary Medicine, Vienna, Austria, [3]Institute of Acricultural and Fisheries Research, Melle, Belgium, [4]Aarhus University, Tjele, Denmark, [5]University of Kassel, Witzenhausen, Germany, [6]Università degli Sudi di Milano, Milano, Italy, [7]ADAS, Gleadthorpe, United Kingdom, [8]Swedish University of Agriculrural Sciences, Skara, Sweden; c.verwer@louisbolk.nl

The aim of our study was to get insight in feather and cannibalism in organic laying hens, its relations with husbandry practices and give recommendations for farmers and policy makers on how to reduce feather pecking and cannibalism. In 8 European countries 107 organic layer farms were visited. Information were collected regarding management, flock, vaccinations, medical treatments, feeding, housing, range management and specific problems. At the end of lay, 50 hens per flock were assessed for plumage condition and wounds at the neck, back, belly and tail. Potential factors related to the percentages of 'hens affected' were analyzed by partial correlation analyses for all continuous and categorical variables. Dichotomous variables were analyzed by means of linear regression. Fifteen percent of the flocks had severe feather damage, 20% had moderate and 65% had little/no feather damage. Less feather damage was found if pre-lay feed was fed shorter, less different feed phases were fed, in case of higher protein and methionine feed content, higher percentage of hens in the wintergarten, higher percentage of hens on the free-range, less often dewormed, lower number of alternative treatments, application of litter replacement or topping, no roughage provided during rearing, offering daylight and no needle vaccination after rearing. Les wounds were found if pre-lay feed was fed shorter, less different feed phases were fed, in case of higher protein content, lower degree of red mites infestation, needle vaccination given at placement, higher calcium feed content and litter topping. We recommend considering free-choice feeding, stimulating the use of the wintergarten and the free range area, litter management to ensure loose and dry litter, provision of daylight and the prevention of red mites. Free-choice feeding is offering the feed divided in for example protein and energy components, from which the hens can choose according to their needs. Moreover, we recommend policy makers to harmonize the compliance of EU-regulations for organic production in the different countries.

Radiographic examination of deformities and fractures of keel bones in laying hens
B.K. Eusemann[1], U. Baulain[2], L. Schrader[1] and S. Petow[1]
[1]*Friedrich-Loeffler-Institut, Institute of Animal Welfare and Animal Husbandry, Dörnbergstraße 25/27, 29223 Celle, Germany,* [2]*Friedrich-Loeffler-Institut, Institute of Farm Animal Genetics, Höltystrasse 10, 31535 Neustadt, Germany; berylkatharina.eusemann@fli.bund.de*

Deformities and fractures of the keel bone are a common problem in layers in conventional as well as organic farms. The aim of this study was to investigate this multifactorial disorder at different points in time throughout the hens' life and to compare the prevalence in different layer lines and different housing conditions. High performing white (WLA) and brown (BLA) pure bred layer lines (Lohmann Tierzucht GmbH, Cuxhaven, Germany) and low performing white (R11 and G11) and brown (L68) layer lines were kept in two different housing conditions (single cages or floor system, respectively). In the 35th, 51st and 72nd week of age digital radiographs were taken from a total of 100 hens and analyzed by an image processing system. Keel bone damage, namely fractures and deformities were found in all lines and in both housing conditions and increased during laying period. Hens kept in cages showed significantly more deformities than hens from floor housing at all three points in time. The proportion of the area of keel bones affected by deformation increased during the experiment in the cage system whereas there was no significant difference in keel bone deformities between the 51st and 72nd week of age in floor housed hens. The prevalence of bone fractures did not differ between housing conditions at 35th week of age. But at 51st and 72nd week of age the animals in floor system showed more fractures than the animals in cages. Brown layers (BLA and L68) showed considerably more fractures but fewer deformities than white layers (WLA, R11 and G11). These results concerning the differences between housing conditions correspond to findings of other studies. Furthermore, our results demonstrate genetic effects on keel bone damage. Digital radiography is suitable for examining keel bones at different points in time and offers a more precise alternative to the palpation which is often used to assess keel bone damage.

Nutritional dietary tools to reduce the incidence of fatty liver syndrome in laying hens
A. Navarro-Villa, J. Mica, J. De Los Mozos and A.I. García-Ruiz
Trouw Nutrition R&D, Poultry Research Centre, Carretera CM-4004, Km 1.05, 459950
Casarrubios del Monte, Spain; Alberto.Navarro.Villa@trouwnutrition.com

The current study assessed the effect of two dietary supplements (FLS-MIX and FLS-LIQ; Trouw Nutrition) that aim to reduce the occurrence of fatty liver syndrome (FLS) in layers. The FLS is a metabolic disease that can potentially reduce egg production while compromising the health status of the bird. Nutritionists have been seeking for dietary tools to reduce the prevalence of FLS thereby enhancing laying performance and animal welfare. Dietary supplements were provided through the feed (FLS-MIX; 10 kg/t) or the drinking water (FLS-LIQ; 0.25% v/v). A total of 288 individually caged Hy-line brown hens (60 weeks) were blocked per BW before the start of the study. The experiment followed a 2 diets (Standard; Challenge [higher starch and energy to protein ratio]) × 3 treatments (None; FLS-MIX, FLS-LIQ) factorial arrangement of treatments. After offering the Standard or Challenge diet during 14 d to induce the FLS, hens were maintained on the same diet but received their corresponding treatment. Laying performance was determined during 6 consecutive weeks. At the end of the experimental period, hens were slaughtered to evaluate the liver status. The Challenge diet successfully induced the FLS as evidenced by reductions in daily feed intake, lay percentage and a greater liver lipid content compared to the Standard diet ($P<0.05$). No differences in lay performance or egg-shell quality were observed among the different treatments, although FLS-MIX significantly increased ($P<0.05$) feed intake relative to None. On birds subjected to the Challenge diet, FLS-MIX and FLS-LIQ resulted in lower ($P<0.05$) liver fat content relative to None (205, 245, 274 g/kg DM for FLS-MIX, FLS-LIQ and None, respectively). In contrast to FLS-LIQ, FLS-MIX decreased ($P<0.05$) liver friability and the presence of necrotic spots compared to None. Results suggest the usage of dietary supplements can be an effective means to reduce the deposition of fat into the liver when hens are affected by FLS.

Hepatic lipidosis: histological and chemical characterization of healthy and diseased turkey livers

D. Radko[1], R. Günther[2], A. Engels[3], C. Leibfacher[3] and C. Visscher[4]
[1]Elanco Animal Health GmbH, Bad Homburg, Germany; [2]Heidemark GmbH, Veterinärlabor, Haldensleben, Germany; [3]Tierarztpraxis Dr. A. Engels, Bönen-Lenningsen, Germany; [4]Institute of Animal Nutrition, University of Veterinary Medicine Hannover, Foundation, Hannover, Germany; radko_dmytro@elanco.com

Hepatic lipidosis (hlp) of turkeys is characterized by a higher mortality and swollen and mottled livers with an excessive accumulation of lipids in the hepatocytes. In the pathogenesis of hlp, infectious diseases (avian encephalomyelitis virus; AEV) or non-infectious agents (like aflatoxins) are discussed as a trigger. Aim of the present study was to take a look at fat content, fatty acid patterns and the iron content of livers in diseased (hlp+; n=12) and clinical healthy animals in the same flocks (hlp-; n=2). The investigations are based on outbreaks of hlp in three herds. Livers from a not conspicuous farm served as control (nonhlp; n=8). The farm size of diseased herds amounted to 10,000-33,000 animals. The complete diets (coccidiostats no longer included) were analyzed for chemical composition and mycotoxins. In livers, crude fat, fatty acid composition and iron content were analysed and histological investigations were performed. Caecal tonsils were tested for presence of Turkey viral hepatitis virus (TVHV). The mortality rate in hlp-herds varied between 1.2 to 10% within one week. Suspicious livers showed a high degree of fat accumulation in hepatocytes with formation of so-called signet ring cells, in individual cases slightly inflammatory changes. Liver fat content differed quite markedly between the groups (g/kg DM; nonhlp: 152±21.2; hlp-:192; hlp+: 394±66.6:) as well as the iron content in the fat-free DM (mg/kg DM; nonhlp: 341±37.3; hlp-:253; hlp+: 1010±258). The ratios between C18:0 and C16:0 were lower (hlp-/hlp+: 0.51/0.24), the ones between C16:1n7 and C16:0 (0.20/0.22) and C18:1n9 and C18:0 (2.42/5.55) were higher in affected animals (hlp+). In one case TVHV was isolated. In diets, DON (1135/1560/<200 µg/kg DM) and ZEA (121/117/19 µg/kg DM) were found on farms 1-3; aflatoxin was not detectable, suggesting that feed was not the primary reason for hpl. The fatty acid compositions in liver tissue were different between livers from groups hlp- and hlp+, suggesting that the acceleration of fatty acid metabolism is deeply involved in pathogenesis of hlp. These changes were analogue to those of a poor prognostic nonalcoholic steatohepatitis in people. Within an infection temporary lower liver iron contents are seen in literature. In cases of massive infections (like hepatitis C in humans), liver damage is characterized by increased iron storage (possibly induced by the virus). In the trend, here the situation is similar.

Sharp decrease of AmpC-E. coli in a broiler parent stock flock

M.A. Dame-Korevaar[1], E.A.J. Fischer[1], A. Van Essen-Zandbergen[2], K.T. Veldman[2], J.A. Stegeman[1], D.J. Mevius[1,2] and J.A. Van Der Goot[2]
[1]Utrecht University, Yalelaan 7, Utrecht, the Netherlands, [2]Central Veterinary Institute, Houtribweg 39, Lelystad, the Netherlands; m.a.dame-korevaar@uu.nl

Extended spectrum and AmpC beta-lactamases (ESBL/AmpC) are enzymes produced by bacteria rendering resistance to extended-spectrum cephalosporins. ESBL/AmpC producing bacteria are found throughout the broiler production pyramid. In the Netherlands 66% of broilers at slaughter carried ESBL/AmpC-E. coli in 2014. The aim of this study is to determine the dynamics of ESBL/AmpC-E. coli in a broiler parent stock flock. About 3,200 one-day old birds were divided into four groups, housed separately. During the study the birds did not receive antibiotics or coccidiostats. AmpC-E. coli prevalence was determined at day 7 (week 1) by sampling 57 randomly selected birds in each group (n=228), using cloacal swabs. In week 12 in each group 57 randomly selected birds were individually tagged and sampled at week 12, 16, 17, 18 and 19. From week 16 onwards, environmental samples were taken in each group using bootsocks. After the rearing period two groups of 30 hens and 3 males were moved to the layerhouse, groups were housed separately. Cloacal and environmental samples were taken at week 21 and 24. In a selection of samples the concentration of *E. coli* and AmpC-E. coli was determined and after culturing a selection of samples was typed using multi locus sequence typing (MLST). AmpC-E. coli prevalence was 91% (CI 86-94%) at day 7 and decreased to 46% (39-52%) at week 12. The prevalence further decreased to 1% (0.1-3%) (week 19) and 0% (0-6%) (week 21, 24). 22 out of 24 environmental samples were positive, even at low prevalence. The concentration of AmpC-E. coli varied between detection limit ($<10^3$) and 2×10^4 cfu/g faeces. Total *E. coli* counts were between 10^4 and $>10^8$ cfu/g. In the AmpC-E. coli isolates only bla_{CMY-2} was detected. The *E. coli* sequence types showed a large variation, suggesting that the occurrence and spread of resistance was determined by plasmid transfer. Results show a considerable decrease of AmpC-E. coli prevalence in a broiler parent stock flock during the rearing and laying period. The concentrations of AmpC-E. coli in the cloacal samples of individual birds were low. However, positive bootsocks were found, even in the absence of positive birds. This suggests that birds were excreting small amounts of AmpC-E. coli, or that intermittent shedders were present. Another explanation is that birds ceased shedding AmpC-E. coli, but environmental contamination persisted, or contamination from sources outside the pen occurred. The sharp reduction of AmpC-E. coli in broiler parent stock in the absence of antibiotics, suggests a selective disadvantage of AmpC gene bla_{CMY-2}.

Link between diet particle size, stomach morphology and incidence of cecal *Campylobacter* in broilers

S.J. Sander[1], B. Üffing[1], M. Witte[1], A. Beineke[2], J. Verspohl[3] and J. Kamphues[1]
[1]*Institute of Animal Nutrition, University of Veterinary Medicine Hannover, Foundation, Hanover, Germany;* [2]*Department of Pathology, University of Veterinary Medicine Hannover, Foundation, 30173 Hannover, Germany;* [3]*Institute of Microbiology, University of Veterinary Medicine Hannover, Foundation, Bischofsholer Damm 15, 30173 Hannover, Germany; saara.sander@tiho-hannover.de*

Strategies to favour gastrointestinal health without antibiotics gain more and more importance in poultry production. It is well known that 'feed structure' influences gizzard and pancreas weight, there is also some evidence that it has an impact on *Salmonella* prevalence in broiler flocks. The aim of this study was to evaluate further effects of diets differing in its 'physical form' on stomach health and prevalence of *Campylobacter*. A total of 225 male Ross broilers (3 consecutive trials) were fed with 1 of 3 botanically and chemically identical diets (day 7-35 of life): a finely or a coarsely ground pelleted diet (FP, geometric mean diameter (GMD): 316 µm; CP, GMD: 468 µm) or a diet with 22% whole wheat added prior to pelleting (PW, GMD: 480 µm). Twenty-four birds per group were slaughtered at day 21, the remaining ones at day 35. In all animals the proventriculus was evaluated regarding the degree of dilatation (none, low, moderate, severe) and tissue samples for histology were taken. Additionally the mass of the gizzard and thickness of its muscular layer were measured. Furthermore, on day 35 *Campylobacter* counts in the cecum were determined by cultural techniques in 15 birds per group. Results While in the groups fed the diets CP or PW, only one out of 75 birds showed proventricular dilatation (PD), 8 broilers in the group FP were affected. Histologically an atrophy of the gastric glands was seen. Interestingly, those birds affected by PD also had lighter gizzards compared with the other ones in the group. As several birds that deceased during the trial showed ascites and PD in the dissection, it can be hypothesized that the so called 'sudden death' regularly seen in the field at the end of fattening period could be associated with PD. At day 35 of the trial 53.3% (FP), 40.0% (CP) and 33.3% (PW), respectively, of the tested birds were positive for *Campylobacter*. Numbers in the cecal content (PW=1.45±2.23, FP=2.64±2.74, CP=2.12±2.78 lg cfu/g) did not differ significantly. Based on the results of Moen *et al.* differences regarding the prevalence as well as *Campylobacter* numbers (albeit only numerical) may be explained by a strengthened barrier function of proventriculus and gizzard due to 'feed structure' (particle size).

Finely ground soybean byproducts in broiler diets: performance, excreta quality and foot pad health

A. Heuermann[1], M. Kölln[1], T. Jackisch[2] and J. Kamphues[1]
[1]Institute of Animal Nutrition at the University of Veterinary Medicine, Bischofsholer Damm 15, 30173 Hanover, Germany; [2]Köster Marine Proteins GmbH, Rothenbaumchaussee 58, 20148 Hamburg, Germany; annika.heuermann@tiho-hannover.de

In broiler diets soybean byproducts are an important protein source. Recently it is on debate whether the main protein sources should be separately ground finely to improve digestibility of proteins and amino acids. The hypothesis of this study was that a higher grinding intensity would improve the performance, the excreta quality, the foot pad health as well as the praecaecal digestibility of raw protein. Three different soybean byproducts were tested, each in conventionally and finely ground condition: low-protein-soybean meal (LP-SBM), High-Protein-Soybean meal (HP-SBM) and Soy Protein Concentrate (SPC). 240 male broilers (Ross 708) were divided into 10 groups at the age of 7 days. The diets were pelleted, based on wheat and corn and the three different protein sources (see above) were used. Each soybean byproduct was available in a conventionally ground version (2-20% of particles passed a 200 µm sieve in a modified dry sieve analysis), but also with a very fine particle size (mean of particles <63 µm; more than 98% of particles passed a 200 µm sieve) due to a new grinding technology. The feed and water consumption were measured on group basis daily. FPD-Scores, based on a modified scoring system by Mayne *et al.*, and the individual body weight (BW) were measured every week. Additionally, excreta and litter samples were collected weekly as pooled samples per group to analyse the DM content. Statistical analyses were performed by using SAS® software (Cary, NC, USA; PROC GLM/PROC NPAR1WAY). The new grinding technology had a significant influence on performance when LP-SBM was used. Regarding HP-SBM and SPC the high grinding intensity did not result in higher performance. But, there was a trend for adverse effects regarding DM content of excreta/litter as well as on foot pad health when only finely ground soy products were used as protein source. The grinding intensity had an influence on performance as well as on severity of FPD, when LP-SBM and HP-SBM were used (grinding altered particle size more marked than in previously 'fine' SPC, e.g.). In a second trial the effects on the digestibility of protein and amino acids were tested. The diets contained either conventionally ground or finely ground LP-SBM. Preliminary analyses showed that the new grinding technology resulted in a higher praecaecal digestibility of raw protein when finely ground LP-SBM was used in the diet (100% conventionally ground vs 100% finely ground). It is a matter of preliminary results, analyses of further groups are still ongoing.

A new floor design for housing fattening poultry to minimize animal's contact with excreta

C. Visscher and J. Kamphues

University of Veterinary Medicine Hannover, Institute for Animal Nutrition, Bischofsholer Damm 15, 30173 Hannover, Germany; christian.visscher@tiho-hannover.de

In Europe housing of poultry on littered concrete floor is the most common and preferred form. The litter offers isolation (towards the floor), binds wet excreta but also allows different activities of birds (scratching, etc.). On the other hand the litter is pervaded increasingly with excreta. More than 95% of the dry matter consists on excreta finally. The continuous contact of birds' feet and skin (not only of the foot pad) to wet excreta is a predisposing factor for development foot pad dermatitis, breast blister and hock burns. Furthermore is has to be underlined that excreta represents organic matter loaded by infective organisms (viruses, bacteria, coccidia, etc.) depending on the health status of individuals or rather of herds in general. Finally it should not be neglected that in the case of veterinary treatment, excreta contain applied drugs, antibiotics and/or metabolites of these substances. Considering the latter aspects it should be intended to keep animals away from excreta as fast as and complete as it is possible. That were the main reasons for the development and testing of a new floor design, called a slatted floor system, that differs in the 'littered area' (100/50/0%) and in the use of floor heating in additional boxes with 100% littered area (G1: floor pens with litter; G2: floor pens with litter and heating pad; G3: partially slatted floors including an area that was littered; and G4: fully slatted floors with sand bath). The slatted floor consists on 'holes' (15×10 mm) and 'bridges' (plastic covered steel; width 3.5 mm). About 30 cm under the slatted floor the excreta are stored during the whole fattening period. The new type of housing was tested up to now in one run with 240 broilers. In this trial with Ross 308 broilers after 35 days of fattening, body weight was quite high without significant differences between the groups (G1: 2,519±259 g; G2: 2,491±272 g; G3: 2,600±256 g; G4: 2,491±254 g). Only one animal died during the trial in G2. The most fascinating result was related to food pad health: At the end of the trial, 100% of the animals had a score ≤1 (according to Mayne), despite of the high stocking density of about 35 kg per square meter. Never before such values were observed in comparable trials in Hanover. In ongoing experiments it is tested whether the 'separation' from own excreta affects also the spreading of pathogens (tested with *Salmonella*) and the development of bacterial resistance. The project is supported by the Federal Ministry of Food and Agriculture.

Effect of floor design in broiler housing on development of resistance in commensal *Escherichia coli*

B. Chuppava, B. Keller and C. Visscher

University of Veterinary Medicine Hannover, Institute for Animal Nutrition, Bischofsholer Damm 15, 30173 Hannover, Germany; bussarakam.chuppava@tiho-hannover.de

Despite all efforts to reduce the use of antibiotics in livestock, the application will be necessary also in the future. Up to now, there are limited data concerning the effect of a continuous contact of animals to their excreta on development of antimicrobial resistance in commensal *E. coli* bacteria in broiler fattening. To evaluate the development of antibiotic resistant *E. coli* under these conditions, different floor designs distinguished in the contact intensity to the excreta were compared. Two consecutive trials with 240 chickens each were performed. After seven days of rearing in large groups, animals were divided into four groups with three subgroups each. In the groups different floor designs were used to establish differently intense contact of the animals to the mixture of litter and excreta: G1: entire floor pens with litter; G2: floor pens with litter and heating pad; G3: partially (50:50) slatted floors including an area that was littered; G4: fully slatted floors with a sand bath. In the first trial, the animals were not treated with antibiotics, whereas in the second trial, once subgroups were treated with Baytril 10% (dosage: 10 mg Enrofloxacin/kg body weigth) on days 10 to 14 of fattening. Resistance of *E. coli* to enrofloxacin (ENR) was evaluated by Micronaut-minimum inhibitory concentrations (MIC; MERLIN, Germany). MIC was determined at day 2 and 21 by sampling 15 or rather 60 randomly selected animals, using cloacal swabs. In addition, on day 9 and 15 litter samples (n=6/group) were collected from two defined locations: the feeding and the scratching area. Enrofloxacin MIC susceptibility breakpoints were used as defined by NCCLS for *E. coli* (≤ 0.25 µg/ml: sensible; 0.5-1.0 µg/ml: intermediate; >1 µg/ml: resistant). In the first trial, *E. coli* from cloacal and litter samples was fully sensible to ENR. Before starting antibiotic treatment also in trial 2, all samples were fully sensible concerning ENR. On day 15, 66.7% of litter samples in G1, 3+4 and 80% of samples in G2 showed intermediate sensibility to ENR: None of the isolates was resistant to ENR: On day 21 one of 15 isolates from cloacal swabs in G3+4 showed resistance to *E. coli*. In the two other groups no resistant isolates were found. Seven isolates in G1, eight in G2, ten in G3 and seven isolates in G4 were fully susceptible to ENR on day 21. The first data from this study provide no clear evidence that there is an effect of a differently intensive contact of broilers to their own excreta at an antibiotic treatment with ENR to the development of resistance in commensal *E. coli*. The project is supported by the Federal Ministry of Food and Agriculture.

A byproduct of swine slaughtering in broiler diets: effect on performance and foot pad health

M. Kölln[1], A. Loi-Brügger[2] and J. Kamphues[1]
[1]*Institute of Animal Nutrition, University of Veterinary Medicine Hannover, Foundation, Bischofsholer Damm 15, 30173 Hannover, Germany;* [2]*Oldenburger Fleischmehlfabrik GmbH, Friesoythe, Germany; mareike.koelln@tiho-hannover.de*

Foot Pad Dermatitis (FPD) is a wide-spread 'production disease' in poultry, whereby the determining factor is the moisture content of litter. Nutritional approaches are needed to minimize the proneness of this disease pattern, not only for economic reasons, but also regarding animal health and welfare. Soybean meal (SBM; the common protein source for poultry) contributes to the development of wet litter due to its high contents of potassium and non-starch carbohydrates. In this study effects of a partial replacement of the common protein source (SBM) by a low potassium containing byproduct of pig slaughtering on foot pad health should be tested. In an experiment with broilers, SBM was replaced partly by a protein rich byproduct of pig slaughter ('swine protein meal', SPM; 65% CP, 19% ash). As the use of pork in the diets of poultry is not allowed in Europe yet, a special approval of the state's administration was obtained before the experiment started. In 2 trials, 4 groups à 25 Ross 308 broilers were kept from the 7th until the 35th day of life. Group 1 was offered a diet without SPM (=control), whereas the other diets contained 4, 8 and 12% SPM, respectively. In this study design the dietary proportion of SBM was decreased from 29.5% (group 1) to 11.2% (group 4). Energy and protein contents in the diets were almost equal, but with a tendency to higher values from group 1 to group 4 (group 1 vs 4: 12.9 vs 13.5 MJ ME/kg FM and 20.5 vs 22.4% CP). Feed and water intake were measured daily on group basis, whereas scoring of foot pads, measurement of individual body weight and DM content of excreta/litter were performed once a week. Statistical analyses were done by using the SAS software (analysis of variance and Wilcoxon-Two-Sample-Test, respectively, $P<0.05$). Increasing dietary levels of SPM led to unfavourable feed intake and weight gains (significantly reduced body weight in group 3 and 4). Although the highest DM contents of excreta and litter were determined in group 4, the foot pad health was not favoured. Remarkable was the observed 'stickiness' of excreta in groups with SPM in the diet. Thus, the use of SPM in broiler diets has an upper limit, especially due to effects on feed intake and excreta quality. Here, the dietary use of 8 and 12% SPM resulted in higher (=unfavourable) FPD-scores. Yet, a combination of plant and animal protein sources seems to be advantageous for multiple reasons (sustainability, environmental aspects), so a different SPM composition (than used here; lower proportion of ash and collagenous material) should be tested.

Enhancing gastrointestinal robustness to prevent major pig and poultry production diseases

O. Hojberg, N. Canibe, R.M. Engberg, B.B. Jensen and C. Lauridsen
Aarhus University, Animal Science, Blichers Alle 20, 8830 Viborg, Denmark; ole.hojberg@anis.au.dk

Rearing robust animals with minimum antibiotic or zinc and copper use, and identifying alternative strategies to suppress infectious diseases like enterotoxigenic *E. coli* (ETEC) diarrhea (piglets) and *Clostridium perfringens*-mediated necrotic enteritis (broilers) as well as zoonoses like *Salmonella*, is pivotal for livestock production. Gastric ulcers are common in Danish grower-finishers (30%) and sows (50%); although no clear evidence of pathogen involvement, strategies preventing ulceration and infectious gastrointestinal (GI) diseases, and enhancing GI robustness overlap. Strategies include use of fermented feed (pigs: fermented liquid feed; poultry: anaerobically stored high-moisture grain), coarse-structured feed (pigs: coarse non-pelleted feed; poultry: whole grain) and organic acids (pigs). Breeding has reduced piglet *E. coli* F4 diarrhea and for F18, the FUT1 gene also attributes susceptibility. Bovine colostrum may improve digestive capacity and performance of premature piglets and contains high levels of immunoglobulins and growth factors like IGF-1; use of bovine colostrum rather than milk replacer for weaners can reduce ETEC colonization and modulate the intestinal immune system. Lactic acid bacteria (LAB) produce organic acids in fermented feed prior to ingestion, and coarse-structured feed supports stomach LAB growth (pigs) or stimulates gizzard HCl secretion (poultry); the upper GI tract pH is thus decreased and the barrier function enhanced, killing e.g. *Salmonella* and ETEC before entering the small intestine. Use of coarse structured feed also prevents gastric ulceration, probably because firm stomach digesta suppresses aggressive component (HCl, pepsin, bile) transfer from distal to proximal stomach parts. Impaired feed efficiency calls for alternatives to this strategy; dietary hemp inclusion can reduce inflammation and increase gastric content consistency, and may prevent ulceration. In poultry, LAB dominate the upper GI tract microbiota; though mostly beneficial, LAB compete with the host for nutrients and some, e.g. *Lactobacillus salivarius*, deconjugate bile salts, compromising lipid digestion and bird performance. In addition to antiparasitic effects, ionophore coccidiostats inhibit Gram-positive bacteria (*C. perfringens* and LAB). Zinc oxide, used in some countries to prevent piglet postweaning diarrhea, suppresses not only pathogens but also LAB; reducing LAB in the proximal GI tract may explain the growth promoting effects of these additives and is important to bear in mind for alternative strategies. Our aim is to exemplify strategies for optimizing GI robustness to prevent major GI diseases in pigs and poultry, enhancing animal welfare and reducing environmental footprints.

Nutritional modulation of the intestinal microbiota: host interplay in weaned pigs

R. Pieper
Freie Universität berlin, Institute of Animal Nutrition, Königin-Luise-Strasse 49, 14195, Germany;
robert.pieper@fu-berlin.de

The porcine GIT is colonized by a highly diverse microbial community, which is increasingly recognized for its role in nutrient utilization and influence on host health later in life. Our understanding of this ecosystem has emerged during the past years but a further understanding of the complex microbe-microbe-host interactions is pivotal to establish successful feeding strategies. Within this overview, three examples will be discussed in more detail. As a first example, protein fermentation in the pig intestine yields putatively toxic metabolites and the inclusion of dietary fiber source may help to reduce their formation. Although this is quite well established, less clarity exists with regard to host response. A few examples are given how protein metabolites and the interaction with dietary fiber affect intestinal epithelial reactions (barrier function, pro-inflammatory reactions) in young pigs showing that a reduction of protein-derived metabolites does not necessarily have beneficial effects for the host. As a second example, feed additives such as probiotics may help to influence the intestinal microbial communities and modulate immune reactions in pigs. Using the example of a commonly used probiotic, *Enterococcus faecium* NCIMB 10415, some recent findings regarding the early-life host immune reactions and the susceptibility to pathogen colonization at weaning are discussed. Third, it is clear that zinc oxide at high dietary level has positive effect on piglet performance and the reduction of post-weaning diarrhoea. This is likely due to the manifold effects of high dietary zinc levels on intestinal microbiota and host physiology. However, a longer exposure of piglets to such high zinc levels may lead to adverse effects on performance and the development of (antibiotic) resistance in bacteria. Based on our current knowledge, the prolonged use (>2 weeks) of high amounts of zinc oxide as alternative to in-feed antibiotics bears the risk of just 'replacing one evil with another'.

Neonatal development of the gut of broilers is influenced by genetics and management

D. Schokker[1], A.J.M. Jansman[1], M.A. Smits[1,2] and J.M.J. Rebel[1]
[1]*Wageningen Livestock Research, Droevendaalsesteeg 1, 6708 PB, the Netherlands,* [2]*Central Veterinary Institute, Edelhertweg 15, 8219 PH, the Netherlands; dirkjan.schokker@wur.nl*

Neonatal development of the gastro-intestinal tract is dependent on an interplay between gut microbiota and the host mucosal tissue. Several intrinsic and extrinsic factors have an effect on the interplay. Here, we demonstrate the impact of one internal and one external factor on gut microbiome development and immune status during neonatal development of broilers. To this end we used (1) broiler lines differing in their genetic background and (2) commercial birds that were treated with a therapeutic dose of an antibiotic at day 1 via the drinking water. In genetically different broiler lines X and Y, kept under the same management conditions, microbiota composition in jejunum was significantly different over period of two weeks between the lines. Furthermore, by comparing the two lines, trends were observed in the microbiota data at the genus level. Different temporal intestinal gene expression patterns of the gut mucosal tissues were observed when comparing the genetically different broiler lines. Birds from line X had higher expression of genes associated with immunological related processes at day 0. Genes related to cell cycle related processes showed higher expression over a period of two weeks in line Y. The early short antibiotic treatment of broilers affected both the microbiota composition in the intestinal tract, as well as the intestinal gene expression over a period of at least two weeks. Significant differences were observed after functional analysis of the mucosal gene expression profiles in jejunum. Especially on day 5 lower activity of immune processes were observed in the antibiotic treated birds compared to their respective controls. To validate these functional changes, immune cells in the small intestinal mucosa were stained and a significant lower number of KUL01+ cells were observed in the small intestinal tissue of antibiotic treated birds. The results indicate that both intrinsic factors (host genetics) and extrinsic factors (short antibiotic treatment) have an effect on the early life microbial colonization of the broiler gut and on the mucosal gene expression profiles. This suggest that also the interplay between microbiota and host mucosal cells is affected by these intrinsic and extrinsic factors. We conclude that intestinal development is a complex process and that both genetic and (early life) management factors influence the interplay between the intestinal microbiome and host intestinal mucosal tissue. Therefore the interaction between genetic background and early life microbial colonization is a major driver of traits on performance and health of broilers.

Secondary plant compounds to reduce the use of antibiotics

R. Aschenbroich and I. Heinzl

EW Nutrition GmbH, Product Management, Hogenbögen 1, 49429 Visbek, Germany;
rainer.aschenbroich@ew-nutrition.com

The worldwide growing interest in antibiotic free production of poultry has led to a rise in non-antibiotic growth and health enhancers in this branch of production. Especially secondary plant compounds (SPC's) come up in the focus. They are recognized as safe and, due to their mode of action, the probability of generating resistances is very low. To show that SPC's can be a possibility two trials are presented: (1) A university trial examined the influence of a microencapsulated blend of SPC's (Activo®) on mortality, weight gain, FCR, foot pad quality and carcass. 1540 male broilers (Ross 308) were divided into 4 treatments (44 pens, 35 animals each, fed a 4-stage feeding plan): control (standard feed), 'antibiotics' (C. + BMD (50 g/t starter, grower) and Stafac (20 g/t finisher I, II)), 'Activo®' (C. + 130 g Activo® /t feed) and 'AB/Act.' (C. + antibiotics + Activo® in the previously named dosages). Significant differences occurred concerning weight gain especially during the last week, Activo® and AB/Act. showed about 100 g higher values and average cFCR (day 0-48, corrected for mortality also was significantly better in the two groups fed Activo®. The Activo® group also showed highest percentage of animals without foot pad lesions (83.64%), the antibiotic group the lowest one (56.09%). Concerning carcass quality the Activo® group showed the highest weights of chilled carcass, wings and legs, the antibiotic group the lowest. (2) A scientific trial was conducted where the blend of SPC's (Activo®) was tested under field conditions. 5,760 mixed broilers (Cobb 500) were divided into 6 treatments (16 pens with 60 animals each). Broilers were raised for 43 days. All groups received a standard diet (starter: 0.025% Narasin, 0.025% Nicarbazin; grower and finisher: 0.05% Monensin). The groups received different concentrations of Activo®: group 1 (control)-0, group 2-100, group 3-130 and group 4-150 ppm, during the whole period; group 5 received 75-100-150 ppm and group 6 150-100-75 ppm in starter-grower-finisher. Concerning weight (lbs; corrected for mortality) all Activo® groups showed significantly higher results than the control group. Feed conversion rate corrected to mortality was slightly better ($P \leq 0.1$) in group 3 and 4. Live weight was highest in group 5 (6.50 lbs) and in group 3 (6.48 lbs) compared to control (6.31 lbs) corresponding to an amount of white meat of 26.46 and 26.44% in groups 5 and 3 and 26.04% in control. Both trials showed that SPC's (Activo®) positively influence performance parameters, but also foot pad health. These results show the possibility to reduce the use of antibiotics by means of SPC's (Activo®) without losing profitability.

Epidemiology, pathogenicity and inhibition of APEC isolated from commercial broilers in Georgia, USA

A. Wealleans[1], K. Gibbs[1], J. Benson[2], F. Delago[2], J. Lambrecht[2], M. Bernardeau[1] and E. Galbraith[2]
[1]Danisco Animal Nutrition, DuPont Industrial Biosciences, Marlborough, SN8 1XN, United Kingdom, [2]DuPont Nutrition and Health, Waukesha, WI53186, USA;
alexandra.wealleans@dupont.com

Avian pathogenic *Escherichia coli* (APEC) causes Colibacillosis, a syndromic infection in poultry. The aim of this study was to investigate the prevalence of virulence associated genes of 3,797 *E. coli* isolates collected from commercial broiler farms in Georgia USA between 2010 and 2014 and to determine the efficacy of 3 Bacillus strains to inhibit the growth of potential APEC *in vitro*. 760 whole intestinal tracts were extracted from presumed healthy birds and sections were collected from the duodenum, jejunum and ileum. All sections were used to isolate and quantify *E. coli* based on selective CHROMagar media. Five *E. coli* were selected per bird for further genetic analysis. A previously defined pentaplex PCR assay was used to screen all *E. coli* for virulence-associated genes (cvaC, iss, iucC, tsh, irp2); isolates harbouring ≥2 genes were identified as APEC. A subset of 580 APEC were screened against 3 Bacillus (B1, B15, B84) strain supernatants to test for growth inhibition. 47% of all *E. coli* assayed were identified as APEC. The most prevalent virulotypes, accounting for 46.9% of all APEC isolates, were tsh/irp2 (11.6%), cvaC/irp2 (10.2%), iss/iucC/tsh/cvaC (9.7%), tsh/cvaC/irp2 (8.2%) and iss/iucC/tsh/cvaC/irp2 (7.2%). The iss gene, responsible for overcoming the avian Complement cascade, was the least prevalent, identified in 24.7% of isolates, while the gene encoding yersiniabactin (irp2) was the most prevalent (50%) with iucC, tsh, cvaC and irp2 present at 31.8, 38.1, 36.1 and 50%. There were significant differences in virulotype prevalence between years: the most prevalent were tsh/irp2 (2010, 12.6%), iucC/tsh/cvaC (2011, 22.3%), cvaC/irp2 (2012, 34.2%), iss/iucC/tsh/cvaC/irp2 (2013, 15.3%) and iss/iucC/tsh/cvaC (2014, 16.6%). The high variation in virulence profiles demonstrates the need to understand current *E. coli* populations, which are likely influenced by host and environmental factors. Understanding APEC virulence profiles in a flock allows the use of targeted prevention and treatment measures, as the these populations provide an underlying risk to poultry health and welfare. Average *E. coli* growth inhibition by the 3 Bacillus were 65.5, 65.0 and 68.9% for B1, B15 and B84. Maximum inhibition was seen for APEC isolates harbouring 3 (B1, B15) or 4 genes (B84), whilst isolates with 5 genes were least inhibited (60.9% B1, 59.3% B15, 60.2% B84, $P<0.05$). B15 and B84 were least effective against *E. coli* collected in 2012 (36.7 and 50.2%), while B1 was most effective against isolates from 2012 (76.1%), highlighting the benefit of multi-strain probiotic solutions for poultry.

In vitro antimicrobial activity of cinnamaldehyde derivatives against the piglet gut microbiota

C. Forte[1,2,3], E. Ruysbergh[4], A. Ovyn[3], S. De Smet[2], S. Mangelinckx[4] and J. Michiels[3]
[1]University of Perugia, Department of Veterinary Medicine, Via S. Costanzo 4, 06126 Perugia, Italy, [2]Ghent University, Laboratory for Animal Nutrition and Animal Product Quality, Department of Animal Production, Proefhoevestraat 10, 9090 Melle, Belgium, [3]Ghent University, Department of Applied Biosciences, Valentin Vaerwyckweg 1, 9000 Ghent, Belgium, [4]Ghent University, Department of Sustainable Organic Chemistry and Technology, Coupure Links 653, 9000 Gent, Belgium; claudio.forte@unipg.it

Cinnamaldehyde, an α,β-unsaturated aldehyde and the main component of cinnamon essential oil, shows potent antimicrobial activities, but its *in vivo* application may be compromised due to its low oxidative stability and pungent taste. For this reason, synthesis of derivatives with the benefits of cinnamaldehyde but without its weaknesses can become of great interest. Cinnamaldehyde and cinnamoyl chloride were coupled to the amine group of glycine and β-alanine to synthesize imines and amides, respectively (GLY-IMI, GLY-AMD, βALA-IMI and βALA-AMD). The chemical structure and purity of the 4 new compounds were confirmed using NMR and HPLC-MS. In 3 replicate incubations, the *in vitro* activity against the resident piglet gut microbiota was evaluated under conditions prevailing *in vivo* in duodenum and ileum. The 4 compounds were tested at equimolar doses (0.075, 0.15, 0.3 and 0.6 mM), with cinnamaldehyde as a positive control (CINN). A blank was used as negative control (CTR). Selective media were used to count total anaerobic bacteria, coliform bacteria, *E. coli*, streptococci and lactobacilli colonies from aliquots after incubation. Compared to CTR, none of the compounds could decrease the number of G+ streptococci and lactobacilli in duodenal and ileal simulations. In contrast, in duodenal simulations, the tested compounds, except the amides at 0.075, 0.15 mM and GLY-IMI at 0.075 mM, reduced the number of coliforms and *E. coli* ($P<0.05$). In ileal simulations, CINN, GLY-IMI and βALA-IMI decreased the numbers of coliforms and *E. coli* at 0.15, 0.3 and 0.6 mM doses ($P<0.05$). Compared to CINN, the two imines showed similar antimicrobial activities against coliforms and *E. coli* in both simulations. Opposite to that, the two amides in duodenal simulations showed weaker antimicrobial activity against coliforms and *E. coli* at 0.075, 0.15 mM doses ($P<0.05$). In ileal incubation, βALA-AMD at a dose of 0.075 mM was less inhibitory against coliforms and at 0.15, 0.3 and 0.6 mM doses, both amides showed a lower antimicrobial activity compared to the other treatments against coliforms and *E. coli* ($P<0.05$). The data showed the ability of the newly synthetized imines to reduce potential pathogenic gut bacteria such as coliforms and *E. coli*, suggesting possible positive effects when given to piglets in the weaning phase.

The effects of medium chain fatty acids after maternal or neonatal administration to piglets

A. De Greeff[1], J. Allaart[2], D. Schokker[3], C. De Bruijn[2], S.A. Vastenhouw[1], P. Roubos[2], M.A. Smits[1] and J.M.J. Rebel[3]
[1]Central Veterinary Institute, Edelhertweg 15, 8219 PH, Lelystad, the Netherlands, [2]Trouw Nutrition R&D, Veerstraat 38, 5831 JN, Boxmeer, the Netherlands, [3]Wageningen Livestock Research, Droevendaalsesteeg 1, 6708 PB, Wageningen, the Netherlands; astrid.degreeff@wur.nl

Maturation and programming of the intestinal immune system in piglets is initiated by early life microbial colonization and is important for the development of healthy animals. A significant contribution to microbial colonization of piglets comes from the sow. Thus, applying maternal nutritional interventions might directly or indirectly influence the microbiota composition and immune competence of offspring. It is not known yet to what extent the effects of a maternal intervention differ from those induced by a neonatal intervention with the same compound. Here, we compared the effects of medium chain fatty acids (MCFAs) as maternal or neonatal intervention on piglets. MCFAs were used for its known bactericidal activity and association with positive effects on (gut) health. Twenty gestating sows were included one week before expected farrowing date. Six sows were given MCFA in their lactation feed (maternal intervention-MI), whereas 6 control sows received regular lactation feed (maternal control-MC). For the neonatal intervention, 2 piglets per litter (n=8) were administered water with or without MCFA by oral gavage (neonatal intervention-NI; neonatal control-NC). At day 1 and 31 of age, 1 male per litter was sacrificed for the maternal intervention, whereas 1 male and 1 female per litter were sacrificed for the neonatal intervention. As read out parameters microbial composition and intestinal gene expression profiles in jejunum were determined in all piglets. Microbial diversity was slightly increased in NI compared to NC, whereas no effect on microbial diversity was seen in MI versus MC. Overall microbial composition was changed both due to MI (10 bacterial taxa) and NI (2 bacterial taxa), although there were no common changes. Biological pathway analysis on differentially expressed genes between control and intervention groups revealed that MI mainly affected fat metabolism in piglets, whereas NI showed changes in immune pathways and metabolism. Again, hardly any overlap was found between the maternal and neonatal intervention. In conclusion, maternal or neonatal administration of MCFAs both affect microbiota composition and intestinal gene expression, but different biological processes in the gut mucosa are changed depending on the administration route. The putative effect of stress due to oral gavage and the supporting functional studies on gut health will be presented and discussed.

Effects of rye inclusion in diets on broiler performance, gut morphology and microbiota composition

M.M. Van Krimpen[1], M. Torki[1,2], S. Borgijink[1], D. Schokker[1], S. Vastenhouw[1], F.M. De Bree[1], A. Bossers[1], T. Fabri[1], N. De Bruijn[1], A.J.M. Jansman[1], J.M.J. Rebel[1], M.A. Smits[1] and R.A. Van Emous[1]

[1]Wageningen University Livestock Research, 6700 AH Wageningen, the Netherlands, [2]Razi University, Kermanshah, 6715685418, Iran; mehran.torki@wur.nl

It has been hypothesized that dietary inclusion of rye would increase viscosity of intestinal digesta, consequently resulting in an effect on nutrient absorption, gut wall morphology, composition of microbiota, and immunity-related processes in the gut wall, and it might be a helpful model ingredient to investigate the negative effects of nutrition on immune competence parameters of the birds. In this experiment the effects of dietary inclusion of three levels (0, 5, and 10%) of rye between 14 and 28 days of age on gut health, digesta microbiota composition, expression of genes in the small intestinal tissue and performance in broilers were investigated. A total of 960 day-old male Ross 308 chicks were allocated to 24 pens (40 birds per pen). Inclusion of 10% rye in the diet did not affect feed intake, but decreased body weight gain, and increased feed conversion ratio. Litter quality was inversely related to the level of rye inclusion in the diet. Providing rye-rich diets resulted in increased jejunal villus height and crypt depth during the first week of provision, whereas the villus-crypt ratio was not affected. During the second week of the experiment, however, the level of rye inclusion had no effect on jejunal gut morphology. Inclusion of rye into the diet did not affect the number and size of jejunal goblet cells. Dietary inclusion of rye did not affect the diversity of the jejunal microbiota, as determined by the Shannon index, although specific microbial strains were affected by rye inclusion. *Lactobacillus* species made about 75-80% of the jejunal microbiota, and rye inclusion resulted in an exchange between the different *lactobacillus* species. At d28, the share of *Lactobacillus reuteri, Staphylococcus saporphyticus* and Aerococcaceae in the microbiota in jejunal digesta decreased with increasing dietary rye. Dietary rye inclusion affected expression of genes in the small intestinal tissue involved in cell cycle processes of the epithelial cells, including proliferation, differentiation, motility, and survival, as well as in the complement and coagulation cascade. At 28 d of age, effects were more pronounced in birds fed the 10% rye diet, compared to birds fed the 5% rye diet. In conclusion, inclusion of 5% or 10% rye to the grower diet of broilers have limited effects on performance. Ileal gut morphology, microbiota composition of jejunal digesta, and gene expression profiles of jejunal tissue; however, were affected by dietary rye inclusion level.

Piglets' peri-weaning intestinal functioning: a multi-suckling system vs farrowing crates

S.E. Van Nieuwamerongen[1], J.E. Bolhuis[1], C.M.C. Van Der Peet-Schwering[2], B. Kemp[1] and N.M. Soede[1]

[1]Wageningen University, Department of Animal Sciences, De Elst 1, 6708 WD Wageningen, the Netherlands, [2]Wageningen UR Livestock Research, De Elst 1, 6708 WD Wageningen, the Netherlands; sofie.vannieuwamerongen@wur.nl

Weaning has a profound impact on piglets' intestinal functioning. At weaning, piglets experience a major dietary switch from sow milk to pelleted feed. In combination with other stressors such as a new environment, this generally results in a low post-weaning feed intake. The resulting shortage of nutrients in the intestinal lumen alters intestinal morphology, which affects the digestive and absorptive intestinal capacity and can impair the intestinal barrier function. This makes the weaned piglet susceptible to infections, diarrhoea and poor growth. To ease the dietary transition, it is important to stimulate early pre-weaning feed intake. In a previous experiment we found that housing in a multi-litter system improves early contact with solid feed and early post-weaning performance compared with a conventional single-litter system. The current study aims to investigate the impact of pre-weaning housing conditions on peri-weaning performance and intestinal functioning. Pre-weaning housing consisted of either a multi-suckling (MS) system with five sows and their litters or housing with individually kept sows in farrowing crates (FC). Piglets were weaned at 4 weeks of age and 2 batches with 4 piglets from 4 litters per system were thereafter housed in 9.9 m^2 pens with bedding material (i.e. 4 litter-mates in 8 pens per batch). A sugar absorption test was performed 5 days before and 5 days after weaning. Via a nasogastric tube, 5 ml/kg BW of 10% sugar solution was administered and 20 min. thereafter a blood sample was taken. Mannitol was used as an indicator of intestinal permeability and galactose as an indicator of active absorption. Pre-weaning mannitol concentrations (nmol/ml) did not differ between MS (1182.7±170.0) and FC piglets (1461.2±120.7). The percentage of piglets classified as 'eaters' on the day before weaning, assessed by the colour of a faecal swab, did not differ between the systems (MS: 87.5±6.1%, FC: 80.2±6.5%) and neither did weaning weight (MS: 7.94±0.32 kg, FC: 7.80±0.33 kg). Post-weaning feed intake did not differ between MS and FC piglets at day 0-2, 2-5, 5-13 and 0-13. MS piglets had a higher weight gain than FC piglets only at day 2-5 after weaning (0.67±0.12 vs 0.39±0.16 kg, $P<0.05$). On day 5 post-weaning MS piglets had lower plasma concentrations (nmol/ml) of galactose (90.9±17.6 vs 157.4±18.7, $P<0.05$) and mannitol (320.1±115.5 vs 591.9±120.1, $P<0.05$) than FC piglets. These results indicate that MS piglets indeed differ in intestinal functioning from FC piglets.

The effect of chestnut tannins on the prevalence of diarrhea in artificially infected weaned piglets

S. Thanner, A. Gutzwiller, M. Girard and G. Bee
Institute of Livestock Science, Agroscope, Tioleyre 4, 1725 Posieux, Switzerland; marion.girard@agroscope.admin.ch

Weaning is a critical stage for piglets which is associated with disturbances in the intestinal microflora and pre-disposes them to development of post-weaning diarrhea. Infections with enterotoxigenic *E. coli* F4 (ETEC) are therefore an important cause of morbidity and mortality in weaned piglets. The continuous use of large amounts of antibiotics in animal production contributes to the increasing occurrence of antibiotic resistance. Thus, alternatives to antibiotics have to be explored. The aim of this study was to determine the effect of hydrolysable chestnut tannins added to a standard starter diet (CP: 17%; DE: 14 MJ/kg) on the prevalence of diarrhea in weaned piglets artificially infected with ETEC. The trial was arranged as a 2×2 factorial design and carried out with 72 piglets, weaned at 23 to 31 d of age. Piglets were allocated within weaning body weight and litter to the treatments and housed as pairs in pens. From the day of weaning, piglets had ad libitum access to either a control (Ctrl) or a 1% tannin (TAN; Silvafeed Nutri P/ENC for Swine, Silvateam, Italy) supplemented diet. The tannin extract contained 45% gallotannins, 9% ellagitannins, and 38% gallic acid. Four days after weaning, 18 Ctrl and 18 TAN piglets received 5 ml ETEC suspension of 108 cfu/ml by oral gavage, while the other 18 Ctrl and 18 TAN piglets received 5 ml PBS. The bacterial strain used was an ETEC (K88ac), LT+, STb+. The groups receiving the inoculum were separated from the uninfected groups by an alley of around 2 m. An oral electrolyte solution was provided to all piglets. For 14 days after infection, the fecal score was assessed daily using a 5 level score (1=dry, 5=watery diarrhea). Once per week the piglets were weighed and the feed intake per pen was determined. In the first week after infection, TAN diet was able to reduce ($P=0.003$) the fecal score compared to the Ctrl diet (2.8 ± 1.29 vs 3.3 ± 1.18) and the number of days the piglets had diarrhea (2.1 ± 2.2 vs 3.3 ± 1.9). However, no ($P\geq0.55$) effect of TAN on average daily weight gain (TAN: 0.4 ± 0.70 vs Ctrl: 0.2 ± 0.27 kg/d) or feed intake (TAN: 259 ± 76.4 vs Ctrl: 244 ± 94.0 g/d) could be observed. At the end of the experiment the infected piglets receiving TAN had a similar average daily weight gain compared to non-infected piglets. There was no difference in the frequency of antibiotic treatment between the Ctrl and TAN group (5.6% of piglets received antibiotic treatment after 4 days of watery diarrhea) and the mortality rate was 0%. In conclusion the tannin extract used was able to reduce the severity of diarrhea but had no effect on growth performance in the first week after infection.

Effects of the extract of sea buckthorn leaf and berry marc on calves with diarrhoea

L. Liepa, E. Zolnere and I. Dūrītis
Latvia University of Agriculture, FVM, Helmana 8, Jelgava, 3004, Latvia; laima.liepa@llu.lv

The study is part of project LCS 672/2014. In previous studies, the influence of the extract of sea buckthorn leaves (SBL) on calves with *Cryptosporidium parvum* diarrhoea (CD) was recognised: TNF-a was significantly ($P<0.01$) lower than in control calves. In 2015, studies were continued with the mixture of SBL and sea buckthorn berry marc extract (SBLM). There was a reduced concentration of tannins two times due to addition of polyethylenglycol. The aim of the study was to find out the action of SBLM in calves with CD and with diarrhoea of nutritional reasons (ND). ND causes were: too late and too little doses of colostrum, poor nutritional hygiene and keeping of calves. The experiment was performed in 2 herds with 265 and 280 dairy cows, in April-July, 2015. In both herds the control (C) and experimental group (E) each consisted of 10 calves. None of 40 calves got medical treatment in the period of diarrhoea. In group E, extract of SBLM was given per os before milk feeding at increasing dosage from 5 to 8 ml/2× a day, starting from the day of birth (D0) till day 15 (D15) for ND and till D20 for CD. Clinical examination of calves was performed every day, but weight gain was controlled and blood samples for biochemical and haematological anaiyses were collected on D1, D10, D15 and D30. In the herd with CD, the number of Cryptosporidia oocites was analysed in the faecal samples of calves every day D0-D30. Data were analysed using computer program SPSS. In the herd ND: in E group, diarrhoea cases were less (3) than in C (5). In E, diarrhoea started 3 days later (on D6) than in C group (on D3). In E, on D10 and D15 the mean number of band leukocytes and levels of serum haptoglobin were significantly lower ($P<0.05$). The level of haptoglobin on D15 in E group was 0.2±0.0 ng/ml, but in C it was 2.3±1.5 ng/ml ($P<0.01$). The mean weight gain on D0-D30 was significantly higher ($P=0.05$) in E than in group C, 453.4±50.1 g/day and 369.9±49.6 g/day, respectively. In group E, the number of white blood cells tended to increase ($P=0.08$) on D15 and D30 compared to group C. In the herd CD, all calves in both groups C and E had diarrhoea, but in E it started and ended about 2 days later than in C. Differences ($P>0.05$) between the mean values of indices mentioned above and in number of Cryptosporidia oocites in E and C were insignificant. In faecal samples of 7 calves in C, unidentified bacteria were found on D0-D11. In E no bacteria were established. In calves with nutritional problems, SBLM can reduce diarrhoea incidence, promote growing rate and reduce inflammation indices in blood. SBLM extract can also reduce bacterial infection in the gut of calves; however, more experiments are necessary to recognize the sensitive species of bacteria.

Pre-weaning growth affects colonic mucosa response to stress long-after weaning

A. Mereu[1], J.J. Pastor[1], C. Dawn[2], G. Tedo[1], G. Rimbach[2] and I.R. Ipharraguerre[1,2]
[1]LUCTA SA, Innovation Division, UAB Research Park, Eureka building, Campus Autonomous University of Barcelona, Cerdanyola del Valles, 08193, Spain, [2]University of Kiel, Institute of Human Nutrition and Food Science, Hermann-Rodewald-Straße 6-8, Kiel, 24118, Germany; gemma.tedo@lucta.com

Weaning-induced stress is associated with intestinal dysfunction and impaired piglet growth. In addition, body weight at weaning has life-long effects on pig performance. Therefore, the aim of this work was to elucidate if variation in pre-weaning growth correlate with differences in intestinal sensitivity to stress long after weaning. To this end, 18 piglets ((LW×LD) × Pietrain) were weighed and identified at birth. At weaning (21 d of age) piglets were divided into two groups (n=9): fast growers (FG) or slow growers (SG) according to their growth rate from birth to weaning. Thereafter, piglets were housed individually and fed ad libitum non-medicated pre-starter (21-35 d) and starter (35-56 d) feeds. Individual BW and feed intake were registered. On day 56 ascendant colon samples were harvested to measure the protein concentration of cortisol, TNF-α, CRH and the mRNA abundance of glucocorticoid receptor (GR), 11β-hydroxylase (CYP11B1), and 11β-hydroxysteroid dehydrogenase type 1 (HSD11B1) in colonic mucosa. Performance data were analyzed with a mixed-effect model with repeated measures in which pig was treated as random and treatment, week, and its interaction were considered fixed effects. Colonic measurements were analyzed using a Student's t tests. Pigs in the SG group had a lower pre-weaning growth rate (181 vs 208 g/d; $P<0.04$) and BW at d 21 (6.0 vs 6.3 kg; $P<0.05$) than FG counterparts. At d 56, no differences were observed in colonic CYP11B1, CRH, and GR between groups. Compared to SG, however, FG pigs had lower levels of colonic cortisol (20 vs 2.5 ng/mg; $P<0.001$) and TNF-α (0.15 vs 0.09 ng/mg; $P<0.01$). In addition, the expression of HSD11B1 gene, which encodes for the enzyme that reduces cortisone to the active hormone cortisol, was downregulated (1 vs 0.68; $P<0.004$) in the FG group. In conclusion, higher pre-weaning growth rate is associated with decreased intestinal sensitivity to stress, which partly may explain the long-lasting effects in animal performance.

Development of an *Escherichia coli* challenge model in weaned piglets

X. Guan, M. Van Oostrum, P.J. Van Der Aar and F. Molist
Schothorst Feed Research B.V., Swine nutrition, Meerkoetenweg 26, 8200 AM Lelystad, the Netherlands; xguan@schothorst.nl

Post-weaning diarrhoea caused by *Escherichia coli* is still one of the main problems in the swine industry. Having a reliable experimental model to test the effect of different feeding strategies against diarrhoea can help the swine producers to ameliorate the problem. For that reason, it is interesting to understand the role of animal genetics in the prevalence of diarrhoea. Thirty-two boars weaned at 21 days entered the trial. The experiment was set up as a 4×2 factorial design with diet (negative control (NC), positive control (PC), higher water holding capacity (H-WHC) and lower water holding capacity (L-WHC)) and animals genetics (Pietrain and York) as experimental factors. Piglets from PC group were orally supplied with colistine. To obtain the H-WHC and L-WHC diets soy hulls and sunflower hulls were added to the NC diet, respectively. During the first 3 days, all piglets were treated with colistine to reduce the *E. coli* colonization in the gut. On day 10, piglets were challenged orally with 5 ml of 8.7 Log of nalidixine resistant *E. coli*. During days 11 to 15, 18, 20 and 22, faecal samples were collected to analyze nalidixine resisitant *E. coli*. On days 8 and 22 blood samples were taken to analyse the acute phase protein level. Outliers were exclude based on the Doornbos test. Experimental data were analysed by analysis of variance as a 4×2 factorial design using Genstat®. Differences were considered to be significant when $P<0.05$. On day 8, faecal *E. coli* excretion was not detectable from all the piglets. On day 12 (2 day post-challenge), piglets from NC, H-WHC and L-WHC diets had similar faecal *E. coli* excretion around 6.5 log cfu/g faeces, and piglets from PC treatment had significantly lower faecal *E. coli* excretion of 3.8 log cfu/g faeces. On day 14 ($P=0.006$) and 15 ($P=0.009$), an interaction between animal genetics and diets were found, York piglets showed the highest *E. coli* concentration of 8.31 and 7.42 log cfu/g faeces, respectively, whereas Pietrain piglets showed the lowest *E. coli* excretion of 3.93 and 3.23 log cfu/g faeces, respectively when fed the L-WHC diet. Acute phase proteins from the blood increased significantly ($P=0.001$) on day 22 (post-challenge) compared with day 8 (pre-challenge). In conclusion, animal genetics and diet should be taken into consideration in order to have a better control of the model.

In vitro inhibitory activities of browse extracts on larval exsheathment of goat nematodes

G. Mengistu[1,2], H. Hoste[3], W.H. Hendriks[2] and W.F. Pellikaan[2]

[1] Mekelle University, Department of Animal, Rangeland and Wildlife Sciences, Mekelle University, P.O. Box 231, Ethiopia, [2] Wageningen University, Department of Animal Sciences, Wageningen University, 6708 WD, Wageningen, the Netherlands, [3] INRA, UMR 1225 INRA DGER, 23 Chemin des Capelles, F31076, Toulouse, France; genet.mengistu@wur.nl

Nematodes impose a significant economic loss in goat production systems in Ethiopia. *Haemonchus contortus* and *Trichostrongylus colubriformis* are the most prevalent species of nematodes. Control using synthetic anthelimintic drugs is limited due to inaccessibility or high cost and tannin-containing forages could provide a cheap and sustainable alternative. The present study examined anthelmintic properties of two tannin-containing browse against *H. contortus* and *T. colubriformis* infective larval stage (L_3), and to compare larval susceptibility to extracts. The larval exsheathment inhibition assay was employed where the L_3 were exposed to extracts obtained from acetone/water (70:30, v/v) extracted dried leaves of *Capparis tomentosa* and *Dodonea angustifolia*. Condensed tannin concentrations were 6.8 and 9.3 Abs_{550} nm/g DM, respectively as measured by the modified Butanol-HCl-Iron method. The L_3 (ca. 1000 L_3/ml) were obtained from monospecifically infected donor goats. Treatments included extract doses of 1,200, 600, 300, 150 and 0 (control) µg/ml PBS. The L_3 were exposed for 3 h, centrifuged and washed 3 times with PBS. Four replicates from each dose were prepared and artificial exsheathment induced using a 40 µl solution of sodium hypochlorite (2%, w/v) and sodium chloride (16.5%, w/v) diluted in 1:400 or 1:500 PBS. Larval exsheathment was recorded microscopically (200×) at 0, 20, 40, and 60 min. Percentage exsheathment was calculated as the ratio of exsheathed over the total exsheated and ensheated larvae. Percentage exsheathment data were subjected to GLM of SAS. The effective dose that causes 50% L_3 exsheathment inhibition (EC_{50}) was calculated using a PoloPlus software. There was a dose dependent effect on exsheathment ($P<0.001$) across extracts with complete inhibition for 1,200 µg/ml regardless of larval species. Mean EC_{50} values were 332.9 and 275.8 (*H. contortus*), and 359.6 and 386.9 µg/ml (*T. colubriformis*) with *C. tomentosa* and *D. angustifolia*, respectively. The extracts exhibited anthelmintic properties against both nematode species and the mean EC_{50} values suggested higher susceptibility of *H. contortus*. Results suggest the possible use of the two browse species for simultaneous control of *H. contortus* and *T. colubriformis*.

Key issues of poultry gut health and microbiota in Nepal

T. Manoj
Agriculture and Forestry University, Rampur, Chtiwan, +977, Nepal; tamangmanoj444@gmail.com

Poultry farming is an emerging industry in Nepal contributing more than 3.5% of the gross domestic product of the country. Poultry gut health and microbiota is one of the most important aspects of poultry management. Maintaining a good poultry gut health and microbiota has been a serious challenge for most of the Nepalese farmers. Most of the commercial and semi-commercial Nepalese farmers rely on deep litter housing system which is one of the major reasons behind gut health issues. Gut health and microbiota is influenced by several factors associated with feed and water. In the context of Nepal poor drinking water, random antibiotics use, unmanaged litter and sometimes poor quality feed are the contributing factors for gut health issues. Enteritis is the preliminary lesion showing the sign of poor gut health. Most of the farmers in Nepal use untreated water exposing the poultry towards *E. coli* and *Salmonella* infections. Many of the farmers have been using antibiotics randomly without recommendations from a qualified veterinarian. Overuse of antibiotics has been another challenge for maintaining gut health in Nepal. Yet another challenge is the feed. The country's dependency on India for most of the raw materials like maize, soya, oil cakes has increased the susceptibility of several mycotoxins in the feed thus intensifying the gut health issues. There is a need of awareness from the farmers' level to the feed manufacturers' in order to correct the problem and get maximum profit from this industry. In the modern times, antibiotics free feed for public health concern has arose another major challenge to maintain gut health and microbiota. Thus, there is need of intense research to manufacture feed that could competitively exclude harmful gut flora to maintain optimum gut health.

Different synbiotic dose feeding effect on the calf digestive channel health and weight gain

A. Ilgaza and A. Arne
Faculty of Veterinary medicine, Latvia University of Agriculture, Kr. Helmana str.8, 3004, Latvia; astra.arne@llu.lv

Looking for alternative means of antibiotics, which could contribute to a faster increase in live weight of calves and their healthier development, prebiotics, are being studied as one of the alternatives. The study is aimed to find out how different inulin dose in synbiotic composition influences the efficiency of feed additives. Depending on synbiotic recipes, we fed 3 different quantities of prebiotics (50% of inulin) and industrially produced probiotics (*Enterococcus faecium*). We formed control group (CoG; n=10) and four treatment groups: SinG6 (n=10), SinG12 (n=10), SinG24 (n=10) respectively prebiotics 6g; 12g; 24g and the same probiotic dose for all groups. Every day faecal mass consistency visual inspection, with the assessment in points 0-3, was carried out. Faecal mass consistency of the SinG6 group calves was evaluated on average with 0.52 poi nts the first two weeks, and then it increased slightly to 0.88 points in the seventh life week. Such common dynamics we observed in other synbiotic groups as well. In CoG control group of seven weeks old animals the results were worse; close to two points. We have stated that in this age a commenced concentrated feeding can cause digestive disorders, which can be significantly reduced by our selected synbiotic feeding. Besides, multiple inulin quantity increase in synbiotic composition does not significantly reduce the digestive problems related to the number of cases. The study was carried out in live weight gain analysis. We found that the dose fed to calves in all synbiotic groups, but particularly in SinG24 group, gave significant ($P<0.05$) increase in the average live weight when compared with the control group of animals (SinG24 0.82±0.151 g; CoG 0.630±0.133 g). Similar, but not so high results in their studies had stated also other authors. Faecal mass microbial inspection showed that with the animal growth, the number of colonies of enterococci increased. Also the studies of other authors indicate that calves in the first 12 weeks of life have the most intensive intestinal canal bacterial proliferation. By analysing all three synbiotic dose feeding effects, we can acknowledge that the samples from the calves, to which the smallest prebiotics (SinG6) dose were fed, showed the same high level of enterococci colonies increase as with four times higher dose of prebiotics (SinG24). Despite the fact that the biggest live weight gain was in calves with the highest dose of prebiotics in synbiotic, the other animal groups showed an excellent state of health and live weight gain. Research has been supported by the National research programme AgroBioRes (2014-2017).

Secondary plant compounds to fight pathogenic and antibiotic resistant bacteria in farm animals

T. Rothstein and I. Heinzl

EW Nutrition GmbH, Hogenbögen 1, 49429 Visbek, Germany; timo.rothstein@ew-nutrition.com

Antibiotics were and still remain the method of choice against bacterial diseases. Due to their additional positive effect on growth performance they increasingly have been used in animal husbandry. But every use of antibiotics imposes positive selection pressure towards resistant bacteria and especially the prophylactic use at low dosage provides bacteria a chance to adapt. For this very prophylactic and metaphylactic use secondary plant compounds (SPCs) could be an alternative as for a number of them antimicrobial efficacy has been published. As SPCs act less specifically than antibiotics, the question occurred if their modes of action are effective against prevalent pathogens but also against their multiresistant variants. For this purpose three trials were conducted. (1) The first attempt sensitivity of diverse bacteria to SPCs was tested in agardiffusion test. The effectiveness of the active substances was determined by the extent to which they prevent the development of bacterial overgrowth. Different concentrations (1, 2, 10%) of a standardized mixture of SPCs and organic acids (Activo® Liquid) were tested for their antimicrobial effects on reference strains of *E. coli*, *Proteus vulgaris*, *Pseudomonas fluorescens*, *Sal. pulmorum*, *Sal. gallinarum*, *Staph. aureus*. Activo® Liquid showed antimicrobial activity on all bacteria tested. (2) In further trial farm isolates of four extended spectrum beta lactamase producing *E. coli* (ESBL) and two Methicillin resistant *Staph. aureus* (MRSA) strains were compared to nonresistant reference strains against Activo® Liquid. In a minimal inhibitory concentration assay (MIC) the antimicrobial efficacy of this blend in different concentrations was evaluated. Result: the efficacy of Activo® Liquid could be demonstrated in a concentration dependent manner with antimicrobial impact at higher concentrations and bacteriostatic efficacy in dilutions up to 0.1% (ESBL) and 0.2% (MRSA). (3) Field isolates of two ESBL *E. coli* and two aminopenicillin and cephalosporin resistant strains (AmpC), were tested in comparison to a nonresistant reference strain against SPCs in a further MIC Assay. Resistance was approved by positive control using cefotaxime as antibiotic. The efficacy of Activo® Liquid could also here be demonstrated in a concentration dependent manner with antimicrobial impact at higher concentrations and bacteriostatic efficacy in dilutions up to 0.1%. In order to contain the emergence and spread of newly formed resistance mechanisms it is of vital importance to reduce the use of antibiotics. The high efficacy of SPCs against ESBL and AmpC *E. coli* and MRSA as well as generally occurring pathogens in farm animals displays the potential of these natural compounds to contribute to facing current challenges.

Dietary supplementation of quercetin improves performance in weaned piglets

J. Degroote[1], Z. Ma[2], H. Vergauwen[3], W. Wang[2], N. Van Noten[2], C. Van Ginneken[3], S. De Smet[2] and J. Michiels[1]
[1]Ghent University, Department of Applied Biosciences, valentin Vaerwyckweg 1, 9000 Ghent, Belgium, [2]Ghent University, Department of Animal Production, Proefhoevestraat 10, 9090 Melle, Belgium, [3]University of Antwerp, Department of Veterinary Sciences, Universiteitsplein 1, 2610 Wilrijk, Belgium; jerdgroo.degroote@ugent.be

Weaning of young mammals is a critical process which interferes with the functionality of the digestive tract. In pigs, weaning is associated with villus atrophy, disruption of the tight junction barrier function and an increased inflammatory status of the gut. It has also been shown that the enterocyte oxidative status affects the severity of these alterations. Therefore, improving the oxidative status could help countering the detrimental effects associated with weaning. To test the potential of antioxidant supplementation at weaning, first an *in vitro* screening of several antioxidants was performed in a porcine jejunal enterocyte cell line (IPEC-J2). Here, the polyphenol quercetin was selected as a high potential antioxidant for *in vivo* evaluation. In this trial, 224 weaner piglets (21 d age; 5.88 kg) were offered a basal weaner diet either containing 0 mg/kg (CON), 100 mg/kg (100QUE), 300 mg/kg (300QUE) or 900 mg/kg (900QUE) quercetin (>95%, Sigma Q4951) during the first 14 days post-weaning. Six pen replicates per treatment were introduced, each containing 7 animals per pen. The animals were allocated according to sex, body weight and litter. Results in the weaning period (d0-14 post-weaning) did not show any significant improvements in performance. However, during the consecutive starter phase (d14-42 post-weaning) a significant higher average daily feed intake (ADFI) was observed in the 900QUE treatment (592 g/d) as compared to the CON (534 g/d), although no quercetin was supplemented during this phase. As a result, also the overall (d0-42) ADFI was significantly improved ($P=0.023$). Furthermore, the overall average daily gain was affected ($P=0.047$), with values of 284, 285, 267 and 302 g/d for the CON, 100, 300 and 900QUE treatments respectively. During the experiment, a select number of animals were sacrificed and sampled at d5 post-weaning in order to determine parameters for small intestinal functionality and oxidative status. First results show a 12% reduction of the plasma malondialdehyde concentration ($P=0.015$) and a numerical deceased jejunal FD4 flux (-26%) in 900QUE piglets, as compared to CON. These parameters suggest that plasma oxidative status and intestinal barrier function were positively affected by adding 900 mg/kg quercetin to the diet during the weaner phase (d0-14), next to the performance improvements.

Effects of nutritional interventions on broiler performance, gut microflora and gene expression

M.M. Van Krimpen[1], M. Torki[1,2] and D. Schokker[1]
[1]Wageningen UR Livestock Research, Wageningen, Wageningen, the Netherlands, [2]Razi University, Animal Science, Kermanshah, 6715685418, Iran; marinus.vankrimpen@wur.nl

This experiment was conducted to investigate the effects of five nutritional interventions between 14 and 28 days of age on broiler performance, composition of the intestinal microbiota, and gene expression in gut epithelial cells. A total of 1008 one-day-old male Ross 308 chicks was distributed between 36 floor pens (28 birds per pen). Birds were allocated to one of the six iso-caloric grower experimental diets (d 15-28), with six replicate pens per treatment. Standard starter and finisher diets were used from d1-d14 and d29-d35 of age, respectively. High level (25%) of extracted rapeseed was included to diets to provide a nutritional challenge. Five nutritional interventions, including a plant extract (quercetin); an insoluble fiber (oat hulls); a prebiotic (β-glucan); an anti-microbial protein (lysozyme), and ω-3 of fish oil were applied in the grower phase. Feed intake of broilers fed the diet including oat hulls and lysozyme was reduced during the first week of grower period compared to other groups, but there was no treatment effect after that. Over the second week of growing period, broilers fed the diet including lysozyme showed increased BWG compared to the control and birds fed diets including quercetin and β-glucan. A trend of increased FCR in broilers fed the diets supplemented by lysozyme was seen during the first week of growing period and FCR in broilers fed the diets supplemented by lysozyme, oat hulls and fish oil improved during the second week of growing period. No carry-over effect on BWG, feed intake and FCR was seen in the finishing period. On d21, hierarchical clustering of the group-averaged microbiota data showed no meaningful effect of dietary interventions based on the underlying taxonomic profiles. Alpha diversity by Shannon Index showed no difference per tissue. A significant taxon-treatment association was found in ileum within genus *Enterococcus*, which was significantly higher in the oat hulls included group compared to control and fish oil, mainly at the expense of Lactobacilli. Principal component analysis on microbiota showed that the oat hulls included treatment was also more separated from the rest of the samples, which were all centred around the origin. Compared to the control birds, the genes related to growth-factor-activity were expressed more in the β-glucan included diet and the genes related to anion-transmembrane-transporter-activity in the quercetin and oat hulls included diet were expressed less. In conclusion, limited effects of dietary treatments were observed on gene expression of gut epithelial cells and the expressed genes seem not to be immune response related processes.

Antibacterial and immune modulating activities of sulfated polysaccharides of green algal extract

M. García Suárez[1], P. Nyvall Collen[1], F. Bussy[1], H. Demais[1] and M. Berri[2]
[1]Amadéite SAS, du Haut du Bois, 56580 Bréhan, France, [2]Centre de Recherche INRA, Val de Loire, 37380 Nouzilly, France; mgarcia@olmix.com

Antibiotics have been used for a long time in pig production to protect animals against pathogens. However, a EU policy has been adopted to implement a sustainable production without adding antibiotics as growth promoters. Marine algae contain in their cell wall water-soluble sulfated polysaccharides with potential biological activities such as anticoagulant, antiviral, antibacterial and immunomodulating activities that are being explored to be used as an effective alternative to antibiotics. A crude extract containing sulfated polysaccharides was prepared from the green algae Ulva armoricana harvested in Brittany region (France) and tested for its antibacterial activity against five strains of bacterial pathogens: *Salmonella* Typhimurium, *Staphylococcus aureus*, *Listeria monocytogenes*, *E. coli* O78 and *E. coli* K88. The bacterial growth in the marine extract in both nutrient agar medium and kinetic continuous liquid medium was used for the determination of the minimum inhibition concentration (MIC). The obtained results showed that this extract was more effective in inhibiting the growth of S. *aureus* (1.9<CMI<3.9 mg/ ml) than those of L. monocytogenes (31.3<CMI<62.2 ml/ml), *E. coli* K88 (CMI=63 ml/ ml) and *E. coli* O78 (CMI=62.4 ml/ ml). Furthermore, the ability of the extract to stimulate the expression of the immune response mediators was evaluated using an *in vitro* cell culture system of porcine differentiated intestinal epithelial cells IPEC-1. Analysis by RT-qPCR showed increased expression of several cytokines including TNFα (8.3-fold), IL-1α (7.1-fold), IL-6 (4-fold), IL-8 (10.8-fold) and CCL20 (38.4-fold). This stimulation of immune response factor expression involved the activation of TLR4 receptor. These results suggest that this extract could be used as a new prophylactic strategy to stimulate the immune response of animals and to protect mucosal tissues against pathogens.

Physiological responses of growing pigs to high ambient temperature and/or health challenges

P.H.R.F. Campos[1], N. Le Floc'h[2], J. Noblet[2] and D. Renaudeau[2]
[1]Federal University of Jequitinhonha and Mucuri Valleys (UFVJM), Animal Science, Rodovia MGT 367, km 583, no. 5000, 39100-000, Diamantina, MG, Brazil, [2]UMR 1348 PEGASE, Agrocampus Ouest, INRA, Domaine de la Prise, 35590 Saint-Gilles, France; paulo.campos@ufvjm.edu.br

Global warming will be one of the most important challenges facing livestock production over the next decades. In such a scenario, pig production will be affected because of the high sensitivity of pigs to high ambient temperatures as a consequence of both their limited capacity to dissipate heat and the high metabolic heat production of modern lean genotypes. In addition, pig production will be presumably more challenged by the effects of high ambient temperatures due to its important development in developing countries mainly located in tropical and subtropical areas. However, high temperature is not the unique factor impairing the sustainability and profitability of pig production. In commercial conditions, pigs have been more and more exposed to health challenges due to intensification of animal production and higher stocking density. Furthermore, the association of high relative humidity and high ambient temperature, that usually occurs in tropical and subtropical areas, benefits the proliferation and dissemination of vectors and/or pathogens (viruses, bacteria, parasites and fungi) resulting in a higher environmental pathogenic pressure. As a consequence, the immune system is activated which induces a cascade of physiological and metabolic responses that, in turn, have usually a negative impact on growth and feed efficiency. Although the specific effects of high ambient temperature and disease on animal physiology and performance have been well documented in literature, little is known about the associated effects of both factors. This understanding may contribute to a better quantification and comprehension of the physiological and metabolic disturbances occurring in practical conditions of pig production in tropical areas and, more generally, in many other geographic areas that will be impacted by the perspective of global warming. Some recent studies suggest that growing pigs previously acclimated to high ambient temperature had an improved capacity to limit the physiological and metabolic disturbances caused by an inflammatory challenge induced by repeated administrations of *Escherichia coli* lipopolysaccharide. Therefore, the objective of this work is to provide an overview of recent research advances (1) on the physiological responses of growing pigs during acclimation to high ambient temperature; and (2) on the potential effects of high ambient temperature on the ability of growing pigs to resist, cope or recover to health challenges.

N-acetyl-L-cysteine improves performance of chronic cyclic heat stressed finishing broilers

M. Majdeddin[1,2,3], E. Rosseel[2], J. Degroote[2], A. Ovyn[2], S. De Smet[3], A. Golian[1] and J. Michiels[2]
[1]Ferdowsi University of Mashhad, Centre of Excellence in the Animal Science Department, P.O. Box: 91775-1163, Mashad, Iran, [2]Ghent University, Department of Applied Biosciences, Valentin Vaerwyckweg 1, 9000 Gent, Belgium, [3]Ghent University, Laboratory for Animal Nutrition and Animal Product Quality, Department of Animal Production, Proefhoevestraat 10, 9090 Melle, Belgium; maryam.majdeddin@ugent.be

Heat exposure has a significant impact on well-being and production of finishing broilers. The involvement of heat stress in the occurrence of oxidative stress has been described repeatedly. The most abundant endogenous intracellular antioxidant is the tripeptide glutathione, for which cysteine is the rate limiting amino acid. Therefore, it was hypothesized that dietary supplementation of N-acetyl-L-cysteine, as a source of cysteine, could improve the performance of heat stressed finishing broilers. Four levels of N-acetyl-L-cysteine; 0 (control), 500, 1000 and 2,000 mg/kg, were added to a basal finisher diet with a ratio digestible M+C to digestible LYS of 0.73 (d25-41 of age). Dietary treatments were replicated in 8-9 pens with 20 male Ross308 birds each. A chronic cyclic heat stress model (T was increased to 34 °C for 7 h, daily) was initiated at d28 of age. Rectal temperature at d41 was >0.2 °C lower for supplemented broilers as compared to control ($P>0.05$). Final BW, growth and feed conversion in the finisher phase were all substantially and significantly improved ($P<0.05$). ADG was 88.2, 92.2; 93.7 and 97.7 g/d, and the feed:growth ratio equalled 2.21, 1.91, 1.84 and 1.80 for the 0, 500, 1000 and 2,000 mg/kg N-acetyl-L-cysteine treatments, respectively. In opposite, feed intake on the treatments 500, 1000 and 2,000 mg/kg N-acetyl-L-cysteine was reduced by 10-12%, as compared to control ($P<0.05$); corroborating previous studies showing reductions in feed intake by excess of dietary cysteine. Mortality was not affected. In conclusion, N-acetyl-L-cysteine improved dose-dependently growth and feed conversion, but reduced feed intake, in heat stressed finishing broilers. Determination of more physiological endpoints will give more insight in the mechanisms of performance enhancement.

Is rumen temperature a proxy of core body temperature in feedlot cattle?

A.M. Lees[1], M.L. Sullivan[1], V. Sejian[2], J.C. Lees[1] and J.B. Gaughan[1]
[1]The University of Queensland, School of Agriculture and Food Sciences, Gatton Campus, Gatton, Queensland, Australia, [2]Indian Council of Agricultural Research, National Institute of Animal Nutrition and Physiology, Adugodi, Bangalore, India; a.lees@uqconnect.edu.au

Body temperature (T_B) is considered to be a reliable indicator of thermal balance. During periods of heat load an increase in T_B is thought to be a reflection of the amount of heat gained by the animal. Recording T_B typically uses data loggers where data is stored and downloaded at the completion of the data collection phase, usually ≤10 days. Few studies have used equipment that allows for continuous recording of T_B over prolonged periods of time. Remote sensing using rumen boluses has the potential to obtain data over prolonged periods of time (≥100 days) with access to real time data. The aim of this study was to determine the relationship between rectal temperature (T_{REC}) and rumen temperature (T_{RUM}) and to establish if T_{RUM} can be used as a proxy of T_B in feedlot cattle. Eighty pure-bred Black Angus steers were orally implanted with rumen boluses. Rumen temperatures were recorded at 10 min intervals over 128 d from all steers. To define the suitability of T_{RUM} as a proxy of T_B, T_{REC} were recorded for all animals at 7 d intervals (n=16). Steers had an initial non-fasted BW of 388.8±2.1 kg. Eight feedlot pens with 10 steers per pen (162 m^2). Each pen had shade (1.8 m^2/animal; 90% solar block). Climatic data, ambient temperature (°C); relative humidity (%); wind speed (m/s) and direction; solar radiation (W/m^2); black-globe temperature (°C), were recorded at 30 min intervals; and rainfall (mm) was collected daily. From these data, temperature humidity index, heat load index and accumulated heat load were calculated. Individual T_{RUM} were converted to an hourly average. Mean hourly T_{RUM} from the 128 d data were used to establish the diurnal rhythm of T_{RUM} where minimum (39.19±0.01 °C) and maximum (40.04±0.01 °C) were observed at 08:00 h and 20:00 h respectively. A partial correlation coefficient indicated that there were moderate to strong relationships between T_{RUM} and T_{REC} using both real time (r=0.55; P<0.001) and hourly mean (r=0.51; P<0.001) T_{RUM}. The mean difference between T_{REC} and T_{RUM} were small using both real time (0.16±0.02 °C) and mean T_{RUM} (0.13±0.02 °C) within the hour T_{REC} was measured. Results from this experiment indicate that T_{RUM} has a diurnal pattern similar to what has been observed from other T_B (tympanic, abdominal and rectal) measurements. Data from this study supports the hypothesis that T_{RUM} can be used as a proxy of T_B. Therefore T_{RUM} can be used to measure and quantify heat load in feedlot cattle.

Performance response of grow-finish pigs to a simulated heat stress under commercial-like conditions

L.J. Johnston, L.D. Jacobson, B.P. Hetchler, C.D. Reese and A.M. Hilbrands
University of Minnesota, 46352 State Highway 329, Morris, MN 56267, USA;
johnstlj@morris.umn.edu

Heat stress of pigs in the upper Midwest region of the United States occurs routinely during summer. Climate change will likely increase heat stress conditions for pigs. Our objective was to simulate heat stress of grow-finish pigs under controlled conditions to document effects on pig performance and provide a model to study mitigation of heat stress on pigs. This study was conducted during winter in Morris, MN (45° N, 95° W). Barrows (n=432) were assigned randomly to one of 48 pens (9 pigs/pen) in an environmentally-controlled barn. The barn consisted of two mirror-image rooms with 24 pens in each room. One room was kept at thermoneutral temperatures (TN) and the other room was maintained at high temperatures to impose heat stress on pigs (HS). Five temperature regimens were selected from southern Minnesota weather records to simulate day and night temperatures observed in a typical summer (28, 17; 29, 18; 30, 20; 32, 21; 35, 24 °C; respectively). Temperature regimens in the HS room were changed randomly every 3 or 4 days. No supplemental cooling was provided. Temperatures in the TN room began at 21 and 18 °C and steadily declined to 14 and 11 °C for day and night, respectively. Day was defined as 07:00 to 19:00 h. All pigs had ad libitum access to water and a mash diet based on corn, soybean meal, and DDGS fed in three phases from 45 to 130 kg body weight. Daytime temperatures in the HS room ranged from 26 to 33 °C and averaged 29 °C while nighttime temperatures ranged from 17 to 28 °C and averaged 22 °C. Daytime temperatures in the TN room ranged from 13 to 21 °C and averaged 17 °C while nighttime temperatures ranged from 12 to 21 °C and averaged 15 °C. Respiration rates of randomly-selected resting pigs (n=8/room) at the end of the study were increased ($P<0.05$; SE=2.75) for HS housed pigs compared with TN housed pigs (123 vs 28 breaths/minute). Average daily feed intake of pigs in the HS room was lower ($P<0.05$; SE=0.04) at the end of phase 2 (2.77 vs 3.00 kg) and phase 3 (2.85 vs 3.27 kg) compared with pigs housed in the TN room. However, average daily gain (0.92 vs 0.95 kg; SE=0.007) and final body weight (129.7 vs 131.5 kg; SE=0.86) of HS and TN pigs were not different. Final backfat depth (21 vs 20 mm; SE=0.58) and loineye area (50.6 vs 50.9 cm^2; SE=0.57) were not different between pigs housed in HS and TN rooms. In conclusion, our model was successful in imposing heat stress on pigs. Pigs housed in the HS room did suffer heat stress as evidenced by their elevated respiration rate and depressed feed intake. However, the magnitude and duration of heat stress was not sufficient to significantly depress growth performance of pigs.

Metabolic profile derangements in heat stressed dairy herds

R.J. Van Saun[1] and J. Davidek[2]
[1]*Pennsylvania State University, Veterinary & Biomedical Sciences, 115 Henning Building, 16802, USA,* [2]*Private Practitioner, Krasna Hora nad Vltavou 231, 262 56 Krasna Hora, Czech Republic; rjv10@psu.edu*

A pooled sample approach to metabolic profiling was used to provide a comprehensive snapshot of herd metabolic status with minimal economic investment compared to individual sampling. Study objectives were to evaluate pooled sample blood analyte concentrations collected at different periods relative to calving between herds with and without heat stress. Blood was sampled from 5 to 7 mature cows within defined time periods to run a pooled sample metabolic profile. Time periods were defined as (days relative to calving): Early Dry (>30 d prior), Close-up (<21 d prior) and Fresh (3-30 d following). Metabolic profiles included urea nitrogen (UN), glucose (Glu), albumin (Alb), total protein (TP), aspartate aminotransferase (AST), γ-glutamyltransferase (GGT), sodium (Na), potassium (K), chloride (Cl), calcium (Ca), phosphorus (P), magnesium (Mg), total cholesterol (Chol), β-hydroxybutyrate (BHB) and nonesterified fatty acids (NEFA). Only data from herds categorized as no problems (NP, n=6) and heat stress (HS, n=6) were compared. For each analyte measured, the pooled sample value was subtracted from a herd-based healthy population reference value and divided by the analyte's standard deviation (SD) for a given time period. T-test was used to determine if deviation was different from zero. Analyte concentrations and deviations were analyzed by ANOVA with main effects of period, HG and their interaction with herd as a covariate. Herds ranged in size from 350 to 650 cows with Holstein and Czech Simmental being the predominate breeds. Herds experiencing HS showed the many alterations in blood analyte concentrations in all periods. Overall HS cows had higher NEFA ($P<0.0001$) and Cl ($P=0.005$) and lower Gluc ($P<0.0001$), Chol ($P=0.001$), Alb ($P=0.0005$), Ca ($P<0.0001$), P ($P=0.024$) and K ($P<0.0001$) concentrations across and within periods. Both BHB ($P=0.025$) and AST ($P=0.037$) were higher in HS herds only in the FR period. Analyte deviation from reference values was greater for HS herds for NEFA (0.39 vs 0.99 SD, $P<0.0001$), Gluc (0.48 vs -0.73 SD, $P=0.0004$), Chol (0.12 vs -0.44 SD, $P=0.0016$), Alb (0.58 vs -0.61 SD, $P=0.0006$), Ca (0.18 vs -0.76 SD, $P<0.0001$), K (-0.24 vs -0.84 SD, $P=0.0002$), Cl (-0.13 vs 0.54 SD, $P=0.016$) and AST (0.68 vs 1.31 SD, $P=0.019$). Analyte deviations between NP and HS herds within periods were different for the same analytes with the greatest differences found in FR period. Results suggest evaluation of pooled samples based on number of SD the sample value deviates from herd-based population reference values have diagnostic potential. Herds experiencing HS show blood analyte changes throughout transition reflecting low feed intake, fat mobilization, hypocalcemia and acidosis.

Early assessment of heat stress-related problem in dairy cows by livestock precision farming tools

F. Abeni and A. Galli

Consiglio per la ricerca in agricoltura e l'analisi dell'economia agraria, Centro di ricerca per le produzioni foraggere e lattiero-casearie (CREA-FLC), Via Antonio Lombardo 11, 26900 Lodi, Italy; fabiopalmiro.abeni@crea.gov.it

Behavior and rumen activity are two main responses for the ruminant under heat stress (HS). We explored the use of their measurement by precision livestock farming tools as early alert for HS detection in dairy cow. The 58 Italian Friesian cows involved in this study (summer 2015) were milked twice daily and fed TMR prepared and distributed once daily for ad libitum consumption. Based on the temperature humidity index (THI), two different conditions were compared on 16 primiparous and 11 multiparous, to be representative of 3 lactation phases: early (15-84 DIM); around peak (85-154 DIM); plateau (155-224 DIM). The dataset for the assessment of the variance partition included all the cows in the herd from June 7 to July 16. The rumination time (RT2h, min/2 h) and activity index (AI2h, bouts/2 h) were measured using the HR-Tag rumination monitoring system (SCR Engineers Ltd.), and were summarized by 2-h intervals. The raw data were used to calculate the following variables: total daily RT (RTt); daytime RT (RTd); nighttime RT (RTn); total daily AI (AIt); daytime AI (AId); and nighttime AI (AIn). The first statistical analysis was performed to compare the calculated variables during the less and the more stressful dates. A second statistical analysis was conducted on raw data (RT2h and AI2h), with day, lactation phase, and time of the day (12 levels) as main factors. A separate analysis was conducted on the whole herd to assess the variance partition of the calculated variables. The date affected AIt and AId evidencing a significant increase of these variables with higher THI in all the three phases considered. Date also affected RTt, RTd, and RTn, evidencing a decrease of these variables with higher THI. The extent of the decrease in RTt ranged from 32% (early) to 37% (plateau) of the value recorded in June. The highest decrease was recorded for RTd and ranged from 49% (early) to 45% (plateau). We did not report cows with clinical disease in the hottest days probably because the RTn buffered the negative effect of the low RTd. The analysis of variance partition evidenced a great contribute of the cow within lactation phase: above 60% of the total variance for AI traits, and a share from 33.9% (for RTt) to 54.8% (RTn) for RT traits. These observations need to be extended to a wider sample (including different feeding management) to assess which kind of threshold could be identified to set an early alert system for the farmer to cope with summer heat stress.

Impact of heat stress on AI and natural service breeding programs in the temperate climate

L.K. Schüller and W. Heuwieser
Clinic for Animal Reproduction, Freie Universität Berlin, Königsweg 65, 14163 Berlin, Germany;
laura.schueller@fu-berlin.de

The objective of the study was to determine the influence of short and long term exposure to heat stress on the CR of lactating dairy cows in different natural service and artificial insemination (AI) breeding programs. Furthermore the relationship between breeding type and parity was determined. The retrospective study was conducted on a commercial dairy farm in Sachsen-Anhalt, Germany from May 2010 to October 2012. The herd consisted of 1,150 Holstein dairy cows with an average milk production of 10,345 kg. The barn was positioned in a NE-SW orientation with open ventilation and a mechanical fansystem. After 35 d post partum cows were treated with a presynchronization program (PGF 2α-14d-PGF2α). Cows that showed estrus after the second injection of PGF2α received natural service by a bull or AI with frozen-thawed or fresh semen. Pregnancy diagnoses were performed 35 to 42 d after the day of breeding. Ambient temperature and relative humidity within the barn were recorded using a Tinytag Plus II logger (Gemini loggers Ltd, Chichester, UK) and used to calculate the temperature-humidity-index (THI) according to the equation reported by the NRC (1971): THI = $(1.8 \times AT + 32) - ((0.55 - 0.0055 \times RH) \times (1.8 \times AT - 26))$. Short term heat stress was defined as a mean THI≥73 at the day of breeding and long term heat stress was defined as a mean THI≥73 in the period from d 21 to d 1 before day of breeding. The dataset contained 5,192 breeding records from 1,537 lactating dairy cows on a single dairy farm. The overall conception rate (CR) obtained was 33.0%. Multiparous cows bred by AI with frozen-thawed semen were 22% less likely to get pregnant than primiparous cows. Cows bred by AI with frozen-thawed semen exposed to long term heat stress were 63% less likely to get pregnant than cows not exposed to heat stress. Cows bred by AI with frozen-thawed semen receiving ≥4 services were 15% less likely to get pregnant than cows receiving 1 service. Multiparous cows bred by AI with fresh semen were 67% less likely to get pregnant than primiparous cows. Cows bred by AI with fresh semen exposed to short term heat stress were 80% less likely to get pregnant than cows not exposed to heat stress. The present study indicates, especially CR of cows inseminated with fresh semen are negatively affected by short term heat stress and cows inseminated with frozen-thawed semen are negatively affected by long term heat stress. The CR of cows bred by natural service were not affected by short and long term heat stress. Therefore climate conditions should be considered in the selection of breeding strategies to optimize AI and resulting CR.

Effect of heat stress on milk production of Holstein cows in Tunisia

A. Hamrouni and M. Djemali
Institut National Agronomique de Tunis, Production Animale, 43 Avenue Charles Nicolle, Tunis, 1082, Tunisia; abirturki@yahoo.fr

The objectives of present work were to characterize the intensity of heat stress to which dairy cows are exposed in Tunisia and to measure the effects of heat stress, using Temperature-Humidity (THI), on milk production and milk composition. The data set for this study was provided by Tunisian Center for Genetic Improvement of the Livestock and Pasture Office. A total 27,126 TD milk record of 3,642 Holstein cows of Tunisia were used. Data were classified as belonging to three regions of the country: Northern, Central and Southern. THI values were calculated using a 5-year period (2004-2008) average monthly temperature as relative humidity data from the regional weather of 7 stations (Gabès, Sfax, Kairouan, Sidi-Bouzid, Béjà, Tunis, Zaghouan). The data were analyzed using the linear model to evaluate significant effects of herd-test day, lactation number and THI. Results revealed the existence of a summer heat stress in Tunisia for 4 months going from June to September. The results of ANOVA also showed significant ($P<0.05$) heat stress effect for milk yield, protein yield and fat yield all studied traits. Milk per cow dropped from 1.2 and 0.9 kg in Central and Northern Tunisia. The milk composition were negatively affected by heat stress. THI was negatively correlated to milk yield (r=-0.1). Milk yield decreased by 0.27 kg per cow per day for each point increase in the THI values above 70.

Evaluation of heat stress conditions at cow level inside a dairy barn

L.K. Schüller and W. Heuwieser
Clinic for Animal Reproduction, Freie Universität Berlin, Königsweg 65, 14163 Berlin, Germany;
laura.schueller@fu-berlin.de

The objectives of this study were to examine heat stress conditions dynamically at cow level, to investigate the relationship to the climate conditions at stationary locations inside a dairy barn and to compared the climate conditions at cow level between primiparous and multiparous cows. The study was conducted on a commercial dairy farm in Sachsen-Anhalt, Germany from May 2014 to July 2014. The herd consisted of 1,200 Holstein dairy cows with an average milk production of 10,147 kg. The barn was positioned in a NE-SW orientation with open ventilation and a mechanical fan-system. Ambient temperature and relative humidity were recorded in 2 minute intervals using EL-USB-2+ data loggers (Lascar electronics, Salisbury, UK) and used to calculate the THI according to the equation reported by the NRC (1971): $THI = (1.8 \times AT + 32) - ((0.55 - 0.0055 \times RH) \times (1.8 \times AT - 26))$. Stationary climate conditions within the barn were recorded on 2 locations within the milking parlor (holding area and rotary parlor) and on 3 locations within the experimental pen (alley, cetral, and window position). Climate conditions at cow level were recorded with climate loggers attached to the collar of the cows within an isolated rubber tube. Sixtyone primiparous and 62 multiparous cows were enrolled in the study. The AT and THI differed significantly between all stationary loggers. The lowest AT, RH and THI was measured at the window logger in the experimental pen and the highest AT and THI was measured at the central logger in the experimental pen. The highest RH was measured at the holding area logger. The AT and THI measured at the mobile cow loggers were 1.56 °C an 2.33 THI points ($P<0.05$) higher than measured at the stationary loggers, respecively. The mean daily THI was higher at the mobile cow loggers than at the stationary loggers on all experimental days. There was no significant difference for the AT, RH, and THI between primiparous and multiparous cows. The THI at the pen loggers was 0.44 THI points ($P<0.05$) lower when the experimental cow group was located inside the milking parlor. The THI measured at the mobile cow loggers was 1.63 THI points ($P<0.05$) higher when the experimental cow group was located inside the milking parlor. Our results indicate, that the actual heat stress experienced of dairy cows differs significantly from the heat stress conditions measured at stationary locations inside the barn. Thus, a wide range of microclimates exists between different locations as well as between individual cows exists inside a dairy barn. Heat stress is underestimated when climate conditions are obtained from one stationary location inside the barn.

Beneficial effect of L-selenomethionine for starter and heat stressed finisher broilers

J. Michiels[1], J. Degroote[1], M. Majdeddin[1,2,3], A. Golian[2], S. De Smet[3], M. Rovers[4] and L. Segers[4]
[1]Ghent University, Department of Applied Biosciences, Valentin Vaerwyckweg 1, 9000 Gent, Belgium, [2]Ferdowsi University of Mashhad, Centre of Excellence in the Animal Science Department, P.O. Box 91775-1163, Mashhad, Iran, [3]Ghent University, Laboratory for Animal Nutrition and Animal Product Quality, Proefhoevestraat 10, 9090 Melle, Belgium, [4]Orffa, Vierlinghstraat 51, 4251 LC Werkendam, the Netherlands; joris.michiels@ugent.be

Amongst different stress factors, the onset of broilers and the exposure of finishing broilers to heat have a significant impact on broiler production. The induction of oxidative stress by heat exposure is described in several papers as well the relation between selenium (Se) and oxidative stress. It is hypothesized that above normal feed Se levels, extra dietary supplementation with L-selenomethionine could improve the performance of starter broilers and heat stressed finishing broilers. Two levels of added Se, 0 (control) and 0,2 mg/kg, in form of L-selenomethionine (SeMet, supplied through the preparation Excential Selenium4000) were added to the basal starter (0-10 d), grower (11-25 d) and finisher diets (26-41 d) containing respectively 0.5, 0.4 and 0.5 mg Se/kg. Diets contained 11.5, 10.5 and 9.5 g dig lysine/kg respectively. Dietary treatments were replicated in 4 pens with 20 Ross308 birds each. A chronic cyclic heat stress model (T was increased to 34 °C for 7 h, daily) was initiated at d28 of age. In the starter period (0-10 d) a numerically difference between treatments was observed. Average daily gain (ADG) was 21.48 and 22.39 g/d and Feed conversion ratio (FCR) was 1.240 to 1.191 in control and SeMet supplemented group, respectively. In the finisher phase (26-41 d) the supplementation with SeMet resulted in ADG of 90.72 g/d versus 87.02 for control group. FCR was significantly improved by supplementation with SeMet from 2.380 to 2.043 ($P<0.05$). Overall (0-41 d) results showed FCR of 1.891 and 1.722 and ADG of 63.50 to 64.99 in control and SeMet supplemented treatment, respectively. Overall mortality was 3.75 and 2.50%. In conclusion, supplementation of broiler diets with L-selenomethionine could be a nutritional tool to optimize broiler performance during stressful periods, specifically during heat stress in finishing broilers.

Effect of Farm-O-San AHS on performance and blood stress parameters of animals under heat stress

A. Saiz, J. Mica, S. Chamorro and A.I. García-Ruiz

Trouw Nutrition R&D, Poultry Research Centre, Carretera CM-4004 km 10.5, 45950 Casarrubios del Monte, Spain; jan.mica@trouwnutrition.com

The objective of this study was to measure the effect of the supplement Farm-O-San AHS on performance (body weight, weight gain, feed intake, feed conversion rate and mortality) of animals under heat stress conditions (35 °C during 4 h/day). The study was executed at the Trouw Nutrition R&D Poultry research centre. The trial consisted of 4 treatments, which varied in the type and level of product added to drinking water: no product, 1 kg/1000 l Farm-O-San AHS, 2 kg/1000 l Farm-O-San AHS or 200 g/1000 l Farm-O-San Vitamin C. One thousand twenty four male Ross 308 broiler chickens were used. Performance (body weight, feed intake, mortality) was monitored from 0 to 36 days of life. Heat stress (35 °C) was applied during 4 h/d throughout the entire experimental period. The remainder of the day animals were held under standard temperature. Animals which consumed the highest level of Farm-O-San AHS or Vitamin C showed higher weight gain, or feed intake ($P<0.01$) than the control animals. The lowest feed conversion rate was found in animals drinking the highest level of Farm-O-San AHS ($P=0.03$). Farm-O-San AHS has a positive effect on broiler chickens performance under heat stress conditions, improving animal's growth and feed conversion.

Heat stress in dairy cows with and without access to shade on pasture in a temperate climate

E. Van Laer[1], I. Veissier[2,3], R. Palme[4], C.P.H. Moons[5], B. Ampe[1], B. Sonck[1] and F.A.M. Tuyttens[1,5]
[1]Institute for Agricultural and Fisheries Research (ILVO), Animal Sciences Unit, Scheldeweg 68, 9090 Melle, Belgium, [2]Clermont Université, VetAgro Sup, UMR1213 Herbivores, BP 10448, 63000,Clermont-Ferrand, France, [3]INRA, F-63122 Saint-Genès-Champanelle, France, UMR1213 Herbivores, 63122 Saint-Genès-Champanelle, France, [4]University of Veterinary Medicine, Department of Biomedical Sciences/Unit of Physiology, Pathophysiology and Experimental Endocrinology, Veterinärplatz 1, 1210 Vienna, Austria, [5]Ghent University, Faculty of Veterinary Medicine, Salisburylaan 133, 9820 Merelbeke, Belgium; evavanlaer@gmail.com

We evaluated the effect of heat stress and shade on dairy cows on pasture in a temperate area (Belgium), using behavioral (shade seeking, respiration rate and Panting Score) and physiological (rectal temperature, fecal cortisol metabolites and milk cortisol) indicators. During the summer of 2012, 20 cows were kept on pasture without access to shade. During the summer of 2011, 10 cows did have access to shade, whereas 10 cows had no access. Shade was provided by young trees with shade cloth hung between them. Climatic conditions outside shade were quantified by the heat load index (HLI). When cattle had access to shade (in 2011), their use of shade increased as the HLI increased. This effect was more pronounced during the last part of the summer, possibly due to better acquaintance with the shade construction. In this case, shade use increased to 65% at the highest HLI (79). In animals without access to shade respiration rates, Panting Scores, rectal temperatures and milk cortisol concentrations increased as HLI increased in both 2011 and 2012. Fecal cortisol metabolites increased with increasing HLI in 2011 only. Shade tempered the effect of HLI on respiration rate, Panting Score, rectal temperature and fecal cortisol metabolite concentration. Milk cortisol concentration was not influenced by HLI for cows that had access to shade and used it for >10% of the day. These results indicate that providing shade reduces heat stress in dairy cattle on pasture during the warmer days of Belgian summers.

The effect of *Allium sativum* extract on pituitary-gonad axis in heat-stressed female mice

M. Modaresi and M. Heidari

Isfahan (Khorasgan) Branch, Islamic Azad University, Isfahan, IRAN, Animal science, No:51, Tohid, Amir Rezaii Alley, Parvin St., Isfahan, 8199813448, Iran; mehrdad_modaresi@hotmail.com

Heat stress is one of the most important environmental pressures especially in tropics which reduce sexual performance by affecting whole vital system. Garlic as an effective pharmaceutical plant has been proposed for increasing resistance against stress. Current research was carried out to study the effects of garlic hydro alcoholic extract on reproductive hormones in female mice under heat stress. Fifty female mice were studied in five groups and ten replications. Experimental treatments were control group (normal situation without receiving extract),0, 200, 400, and 800 mg/kg of body weight of extract for thirty days in term of 4 h daily heat stress. Blood samples were taken at the end of experiment period and estrogen, progesterone, FSH and LH hormones were measured. Obtained data were analyzed using SPSS program. Heat stress reduced all sexual hormones significantly ($P<0.05$) in zero group but FSH and LH amount were increased by 400 and 800 mg/kg doses. Estrogen and progesterone amounts were increased significantly in 200, 400, and 800 mg/kg groups and were about control group. Considering the results, extract can be effective under heat stress and neutralize negative effects of stress by affecting pituitary; gonadal axis and ovarian secretion.

Influence of environmental temperature on the reproductive ability of Holstein cows

S. Doroshchuk[1], I. Shapiev[2] and E. Nikitkina[2]
[1]PZ Krasnoarmejskij, Gromovo, 188740 Leningrad region, Russian Federation, [2]All-Russia research institute of farm animal genetics and breeding, Moscowskoye sh. 55-a, 196625 St. Pereburg, Russian Federation; nikitkinae@yandex.ru

High milk production often causes infertility in dairy cows. Cows with high milk production sometimes don't show the signs of the estrus and they have reduced estrus period. All of these complicates accurate determination of the cows in heat. One of the factors that have a negative impact on the reproductive ability and productivity in dairy cattle is seasonal temperature changes. This is especially true for high temperature and humidity. Increased temperature changes in the summer is a stress factor that leads to growth of lipid peroxidation and disruption of the physiological processes at the subcellular level. Violation in estrus cycle, maturation of gametes, reduced fertility increase in dairy cattle especially, in cows with high milk. We studied the effect of increasing of air temperature on the reproductive ability of cows. The study was conducted in June and July. Air temperature varied from 9 to 26 °C (average 15 °C) in June and from 22 to 31 °C (average 26 °C) in July. 167 Holstein heifers and 199 dairy cows with average milk yield 8,895±77.5 were used. AI was performed after heat detection by Heatime HR. First insemination pregnancy rate was 23.8% (cows) and 70.5% (heifers) in June, 18.1% (cows) and 29% (heifers) in July. Total pregnancy rate: 50.5% (cows) and 97.4% (heifers), 41.5% (cows) and 60% (heifers) respectively. Open days period in cows was 129±8,1 days in June and 142±12,5 days in July. It was found that increasing of temperature has a significant negative effect on the reproductive ability of cows and heifers. This heifers are more susceptible to the adverse effects of increased temperature than cows. Antioxidants reduce the negative effect of stress factors and development of peroxidation. One of these antioxidants is Dihydroquercetin (Taxifolin). Adding of Dihydroquercetin to nutrition provided antioxidant protection and helped to reduce negative effect on the reproductive ability in dairy cows under high temperature stress.

Effect of selenium on the growth performance and antioxidant status of stressed broiler birds

B.C. Amaefule, I.E. Uzochukwu and M.C. Ezeokonkwo
University of Nigeria, Department of Animal Science, Nsukka, 410101 Nigeria;
bright.amaefule@unn.edu.ng

The study was designed to evaluate the effect of dietary selenium (Se) supplementation on the growth performance, lipid peroxidation, and anti-oxidative status of broiler birds exposed to oxidative stress induced by synthetic glucocorticoid, dexamethasone (DEX) injection. One hundred and twenty (120) five-weeks-old broiler finishers of Anak strain were used for the study in a completely randomized design (CRD). The birds were randomly divided into 4 treatment groups: T1 (no Se, no DEX) which served as the control, T2 (DEX 4 mg/bird/day+0.15 mg Se/kg diet), T3 (DEX 4 mg/bird/day+0.30 mg Se/kg diet), and T4 (DEX 4 mg/bird/day). Each treatment was replicated 3 times with 10 birds per replicate. Treatments lasted for 7 days at the end of which blood samples were collected for laboratory analysis. Results showed that oxidative stress induced by injection of DEX (4 mg/bird/d) resulted in poor growth performance and lowered antioxidant status. The final body weight (FBW), body weight gain (BWG), feed intake (FI) and feed conversion ratio (FCR) were significantly ($P<0.05$) improved with increasing dietary selenium levels. The mean ± SEM for T1, T2, T3, and T4 groups for BWG were 1.39±0.29, 0.87±0.35, 0.97±0.18, and 0.66±0.16; and for FCR were 2.87±0.82, 3.53±0.12, 3.21±0.48, and 3.99±0.94 respectively. Also, there were significant ($P<0.05$) differences in the blood levels of catalase enzyme activity, superoxide dismutase (SOD), serum selenium concentration and glutathione peroxidase activity, which were lowest in the T4 and appeared to increase as the levels of dietary Se increased. However, birds in the control and Se treated group showed lower malondialdehyde (MDA) than those of the DEX alone. mean ± SEM values for blood Se and MDA levels were 1.83±0.25, 2.60±0.40, 2.68±0.39, and 1.63±0.23; and 1.35±0.01, 1.24±0.01, 1.16±0.02, and 1.22±0.01 for T1, T2, T3, and T4 respectively. It was concluded from the study that supplementation of selenium at 0.3 mg/kg diet enhanced growth performance and anti-oxidative status of broiler birds under stressed conditions without negative effects; which could be useful in ameliorating the effect of oxidative stress resulting commonly from heat and other common forms of stress prominent in the sub-tropical regions.

Prevention of hypocalcemia in periparturient dairy cows: the key role of serotonin

L.E. Hernández-Castellano[1], L.L. Hernandez[2], S. Weaver[2] and R.M. Bruckmaier[1]
[1]Vetsuisse Faculty University of Bern, Veterinary Physiology, Bremgartenstrasse 109a, 3001, Switzerland, [2]University of Wisconsin, Department of Dairy Science, Observatory Drive, 53706, USA; lorenzo.hernandez@vetsuisse.unibe.ch

During the periparturient period, dairy cows are often not able to maintain adequate blood Ca^{2+} concentrations due to the mammary gland's sudden high demand for Ca^{2+}. Hypocalcemia impacts animal health, production, and welfare. Serotonin (5-HT) has been shown to be a key factor to induce the mobilization of Ca^{2+} from bones. Therefore, we hypothesized that administration of 5-hydroxy-L-Tryptophan (5-HTP), a 5-HT precursor, can increase 5-HT concentration in blood, and in turn induce Ca^{2+} mobilization from bone. In this study, 20 Holstein dairy cows were randomly assigned to two experimental groups. Ten animals received a daily i.v. infusion of one liter of 0.9% NaCl containing 1 mg of 5-HTP/kg BW. The other 10 animals received one liter of 0.9% NaCl daily (control; C). Infusions were performed beginning on day 10 before the estimated parturition. Infusions were conducted until the day of parturition, resulting in at least 4 days of infusion. Until parturition, blood samples were collected every morning before the infusions, and after parturition daily until day 7, and on day 30. Milk yield was recorded during this period. No differences between groups were observed for blood glucose, Mg^{2+}, beta-hydroxybutyrate, and non-esterified fatty acid concentrations. Serum Ca^{2+} concentrations decreased in both groups around parturition ($P<0.05$), however, the 5-HTP group had higher blood Ca^{2+} concentrations than controls on day 1 (1.93 ± 0.06 vs 1.62 ± 0.09 mM) and day 2 (2.07 ± 0.04 vs 1.83 ± 0.07 mM), respectively ($P<0.05$). Interestingly, three cows showed clinical hypocalcemia after calving, all from the C group. In addition, colostrum yield was lower in the 5-HTP group compared to the C group (5.63 ± 0.34 vs 8.56 ± 0.47 kg; $P<0.05$), however no differences in colostrum IgG concentration were detected (68.41 ± 5.20 vs 60.70 ± 10.27 mg/ml; $P>0.05$). Milk yield did not differ between groups during the rest of the experiment. Serum 5-HT concentration was increased until day 5 after partum in the 5-HTP group compared to the C group. Similarly, 5-HT concentration in colostrum was higher in the 5-HTP group than in the control one (37.10 ± 3.12 vs 25.02 ± 2.75 nM; $P<0.05$), however no differences were detected in milk 7 days after partum (13.43 ± 1.12 vs 14.63 ± 1.13 nM; $P>0.05$). In conclusion, 5-HTP can reduce the decline in blood Ca^{2+} concentration around parturition, and hence the occurrence of clinical or subclinical hypocalcemia. Additionally, 5-HTP appears to reduce colostrum production, even colostrum yield is still more than sufficient to fulfill the needs of the offspring.

A metabolomics approach to characterize metabolic phenotypes in periparturient dairy cows

Á. Kenéz[1], S. Dänicke[2], M. Von Bergen[3] and K. Huber[1]
[1]University of Hohenheim, Institute of Animal Science, Fruwirthstr. 35, 70599 Stuttgart, Germany, [2]'Friedrich-Loeffler-Institut' Federal Research Institute for Animal Health, Institute of Animal Nutrition, Bundesallee 50, 38116 Braunschweig, Germany, [3]Helmholtz Centre for Environmental Research, Department of Metabolomics, Permoserstr. 15, 04318 Leipzig, Germany; akos.kenez@uni-hohenheim.de

High-yielding dairy cows experience great metabolic stress during the transition from late pregnancy to early lactation. This is due to the complex adaptation processes affecting energy homeostasis in support of milk production. According to their adaptation efficiency some cows develop severe metabolic diseases while others are able to maintain metabolic health. This study aimed to characterise metabolic pathways affected the most during the transition period, and to identify individual metabotypes within the cow population. Twenty-six German Holstein cows were used to collect blood samples repeatedly during the transition period: 42 and 10 days before calving and 3, 21 and 100 days after calving. Blood serum samples were subjected to a targeted liquid chromatography-mass spectrometry (LC-MS) based metabolomics analysis using the AbsoluteIDQ® p180 Kit of Biocrates Life Science AG (Innsbruck, Austria). Processed metabolomics data were evaluated by principal component analysis (PCA) and by heatmap visualisation. The PCA revealed a clear separation of the blood samples according to the sampling day, indicating a notable shift of the metabolic composition during the studied period. According to the complex heatmap the acylcarnitines provided a clear and consistent separation of cows within the herd. The concentration of glycerophospholipids and sphingolipids was remarkably decreased 10 day before and 3 days after calving than earlier and later in the transition period. Amino acids and biogenic amines showed a more homogenous pattern with less variation in concentrations over time. Analysing longitudinal changes of the blood metabolome and identifying new biomarkers by this approach can help understanding the multifaceted metabolic adaptation of transition dairy cows. The biological interpretation of the differences in blood acylcarnitine concentration may serve as a source for characterizing and predicting healthy and diseased metabolic phenotypes in dairy cows.

Association of peripartum serum retinol with metabolic, Inflammatory, and oxidative stress in cows

T.H. Herdt, B. Norby, J. Gandy and L.M. Sordillo
Michigan State University, Large Animal Clinical Sciences, Wilson Rd., East Lansing Michigan, 48824, USA; herdt@msu.edu

The long-term goal is to evaluate serum retinol as a component of a multivariate index of disease risk in prepartum dairy cows. The immediate objective was to determine the relationship of serum retinol to other indices of metabolic stress. Cows (260) distributed across 5 herds were sampled at -48±12 days (dry off), -15±7(precalving), and 7±3 (fresh) days relative to calving. Herds selected had excellent production and management with diets meeting NRC requirements for vitamin A and other nutrients. A step-down regression analysis with serum retinol as the dependent variable was carried out for each sampling time. Initial independent variables included serum concentrations of NEFA, albumin, cholesterol, alpha amyloid, haptoglobin, and antioxidant potential. Additional variables included lactation number, interval from sampling to calving, and farm. A significant ($P<0.001$) portion of serum retinol variability was explained by the model at each time point, with R^2 values of 0.29, 0.55, and 0.69 at the dry off, precalving, and fresh time points, respectively. All of the serum variables remained in the model at the precalving and fresh time points while albumin and haptoglobin were the only serum variables in the model at dry off. Farm remained in the model at all times, however when farm was deleted, the respective R^2 values were not substantially reduced (0.24, 0.42, and 0.58, $P<0.001$), indicating that at cow-level the association is robust with respect to environmental and dietary effects. Metabolic, inflammatory, and oxidative stresses are known to increase throughout the period of lactogenesis and early lactation. Across this time period, as observed in this study, the progressive increase in the association of serum retinol with known predictors of metabolic, inflammatory, and/or oxidative stress suggests these stressors affect serum retinol. Most modern dairy cows are fed adequate amounts of vitamin A and their livers are expected to contain ample vitamin A reserves. Serum retinol concentrations are thus expected to be more a reflection of the liver's ability to mobilize vitamin A than of its vitamin A reserves. Mobilization of vitamin A and the associated increase in serum retinol concentrations requires the synthesis of retinol binding protein, which is known to be adversely affected by inflammation and negative protein balance. We interpret the results of this experiment to suggest that serum retinol may have utility in assessing the metabolic and inflammatory stresses on cows, and thus may be useful in the construction of a multivariate index of disease risk.

Relationship between adiponectin concentration, BCS and insulin response in dry dairy cows

J. De Koster[1], C. Urh[2], H. Sauerwein[2] and G. Opsomer[1]
[1]Faculty of Veterinary Medicine Ghent University, Department of Reproduction Obstetrics and Herd Health, salisburylaan 133, 9820 Merelbeke, Belgium, [2]Institute for Animal Science University of Bonn, Physiology and Hygiene Unit, Katzenburgweg 7-9, 53115 Bonn, Germany; geert.opsomer@ugent.be

In dairy cows, excessive BCS is a risk factor for an increased state of insulin resistance and has been related with several pathological conditions. In humans, adiponectin is negatively associated with the amount of adipose tissue and exerts insulin sensitizing effects. Purpose was to describe relationship between adiponectin concentration, BCS and insulin response of glucose and NEFA metabolism in dry dairy cows. Nine healthy dairy cows with a varying BCS (3 to 5), were followed from the beginning of the dry period by weekly blood sampling and assessment of BCS. Hyperinsulinemic euglycemic clamp tests were performed consisting of 4 insulin infusions (0.1; 0.5; 2;5 mU/kg/min). Blood glucose level was determined regularly using a glucometer and a glucose infusion was adapted to keep glucose level constant during the steady state. Glucose infusion rate, NEFA and insulin concentration during steady state were used to create dose response curves and to determine insulin sensitivity (insulin concentration needed to elicit halfmaximal effect;EC50),insulin responsiveness of the glucose (maximal stimulatory effect of insulin;$max_{glucose}$) and NEFA (maximal inhibitory effect of insulin;min_{NEFA}) metabolism. Serum adiponectin concentration was determined using a bovine specific ELISA. Effect of BCS and time during the dry period on adiponectin concentrations was determined using linear mixed models. To determine the effect of adiponectin on parameters derived from dose response curves, Pearson correlation coefficients were calculated. Adiponectin concentration during the dry period ranged from 19.6 to 42.6 µg/ml and was negatively related with the BCS ($P<0.05$). Concentration of adiponectin dropped at the end of the dry period ($P<0.05$). Insulin sensitivity of the glucose ($EC50_{glucose}=76.4\pm13.4$ µU/ml) and NEFA ($EC50_{NEFA}=19.4\pm4.4$ µU/ml) metabolism were not related to the average adiponectin concentration during the dry period ($r=-0.2$; $P>0.05$ and $r=-0.1$;$P>0.05$). Insulin responsiveness of the glucose ($max_{glucose}=18.5\pm1.3$ µmol/kg/min) and NEFA ($min_{NEFA}=9.9\pm2.0$%) metabolism were positively ($r=0.8$; $P<0.05$) and negatively ($r=-0.7$; $P<0.05$) related to the average adiponectin concentration. In dairy cows, adiponectin concentration during the dry period is negatively related with BCS and decreases at the end of the dry period. Average adiponectin concentration during the dry period has a positive effect on insulin's maximal stimulatory or inhibitory effect on the glucose and NEFA metabolism while no relation was found with insulin sensitivity.

Customising dry period length to improve adaptation to lactation in dairy cows

A.T.M. Van Knegsel[1], N. Mayasari[1], J. Chen[1], R. Van Hoeij[1], A. Kok[1,2] and B. Kemp[1]
[1]Wageningen University, Adaptation Physiology group, De Elst 1, 6708 WD Wageningen, the Netherlands, [2]Wageningen University, Animal Production Systems group, De Elst 1, 6708 WD Wageningen, the Netherlands; ariette.vanknegsel@wur.nl

The high disease incidence in dairy cows during early lactation has been attributed to the high metabolic priority for lactation and an inability to adapt effectively to lactation. Moreover, several metabolic diseases and disorders in early lactation are related with management of the cow during the period before calving, especially the dry period. Recently, we focused in several studies on determining the value of shorter dry periods to improve adaptation to the next lactation. These studies focused in particular on the energy balance and related metabolites in early lactation, calf health, and long term effects, including lactation persistency and consequences in successive lactations. Results of these studies indicate that shortening and omitting the dry period shift milk yield from the critical period shortly after calving to the period before calving, when energy needs can be met easily. Differences in milk yield and health indicators between cows with different dry period lengths were significant. Shortening the dry period from 60 to 30 days resulted in a limited reduction in milk yield, but improved the energy balance in the subsequent lactation and had no consequences for somatic cell count in milk, colostrum quality, or development of the calves. Omitting the dry period resulted in a strong reduction in milk yield, but also had a large positive impact on the energy balance, metabolic status and ovarian cyclicity in the subsequent lactation. Omitting the dry period decreased antibody titers in colostrum and in plasma of the calves in the first weeks of life, but had no long-term consequences on calf development. Cows with no dry period had an increased risk of fattening in late lactation. Effects of dry period length on lactation persistency were absent. Milk yield losses, but also improvement of the energy balance, after a short or no dry period were reduced when this management strategy was applied over successive lactations. Effects of a short or no dry period on milk yield and energy balance were dependent on parity, genotype, body condition score and udder health status. Studies are ongoing to determine cow characteristics that are related to the individual cow response to a short or no dry period. These studies aim at the development of a decision support tool for dry period length and use of dry cow antibiotics, in order to optimize management of individual cows. This 'Customised Dry Period' will not only be evaluated for consequences on cow health and productivity, but also for the effects on net herd returns and environmental impacts.

Extended lactation: an option to improve fertility and productivity in high-yielding dairy cows

M. Kaske[1], G. Niozas[2], P. Baling[3], T. Wagner[3], S. Wiedemann[4], M. Feldmann[1], H. Bollwein[1] and G. Tsousis[5]
[1]*Vetsuissse Faculty Zurich, Departement for Farm Animals, Winterthurerstrasse 260, 8057 Zurich, Switzerland,* [2]*University for Veterinary Medicine, Clinic for Cattle, Bischofsholer Damm 15, 30173 Hannover, Germany,* [3]*Agrar Milchviehanlage Ruppendorf, Bergstrasse, 01744 Dippoldiswalde, Germany,* [4]*Rhine-Waal University of Applied Sciences, Life Sciences, Marie-Curie-Straße 1, 47533 Kleve, Germany,* [5]*Aristotle University of Thessaloniki, Clinic of Farm Animals, Stavrou Voutyra Street, Thessaloniki 541 24, Greece; martin.kaske@web.de*

It was the objective to investigate whether a substantial elongation of the 305 d lactation period (LP) represents a useful tool for high-yielding dairy herds to improve fertility, productivity and herd health. A prospective field study took place on a large dairy (1,092 cows, 11,488 kg milk/305 d) in Saxony/Germany. On day 40 post partum, (p.p.) all cows were clinically investigated and transrectal sonography was performed. Cows without pathologic findings were randomly allocated to groups of cows with a voluntary waiting period (VWP) of either 40 d (VWP40, n=136), 120 d (VWP120, n=135) or 180 d (VWP180, n=132). Cows observed in estrus within 40 d after the end of the respective VWP were inseminated; an Ovsynch-protocol was applied for all remaining cows. A pregnancy check was performed 40 d after insemination. Backfat thickness was assessed prior to next calving sonographically. Frequent recordings of milk yield and constituents allowed to calculate lactational milk yield. Results showed that more inseminations were required in cows of VWP 40 compared to VWP120 and VWP180 (1.8 vs 1.6 vs 1.5; $P<0.05$). Conception rate after first insemination was 36.3% in VWP40 cows; this was lower ($P<0.05$) than in VWP120 (49.6%) and in VWP 180 (50.0%). Ovsynch protocols had to be performed in 30.3% of VWP40 cows but only in 11.1 and 9.1% of the cows in VWP120 and VWP180. Energy-corrected milk yield was 12,025 kg in VWP40 cows within a LP of 346 d (calving interval [CI] 393 d), 13,840 kg in VWP120 cows (LP 396 d, CI 447 d) and 15,454 kg in VWP180 cows (LP 442 d, 497 d). Accordingly, ECM yield per day of lactation did not differ between the groups (34.8 vs 34.9 vs 34.9 kg/d). Persistency was superior in VWP120 and VWP180 cows as reflected by a significantly higher ECM yield within 305 d p.p. in VWP120 (11,334 kg) and VWP180 cows (11,707 kg) compared to VWP40 cows (10,892 kg). Neither somatic cell count nor body condition prior to next calving were affected by the duration of the LP. It is concluded that a LP of up to 500 days may be useful for farms with a high milk yield and a superior feeding management. Moreover, it is suggested to calculate in future expenses for fertility not per cow per lactation but per 10,000 kg ECM produced.

Production diseases 2.0: surplus or lack of nutrients in transition dairy cows?

J.J. Gross and R.M. Bruckmaier
Veterinary Physiology, Vetsuisse Faculty University of Bern, Bremgartenstrasse 109a, 3012 Bern,
Switzerland; josef.gross@vetsuisse.unibe.ch

Beta-hydroxybutyrate (BHBA) representing the most prominent circulating ketone body in ruminants can be considered as energy source for some tissues, especially during a negative energy balance. However, an elevation of plasma BHBA concentration above 1.2 mmol/l indicates subclinical ketosis in dairy cows with detrimental effects on animal health, performance and fertility. The elevation of plasma BHBA concentration impairs glucose metabolism, and increased the risk of clinical ketosis, displaced abomasum, metritis and subsequent decrease of milk production. Recent studies could proof for the first time in dairy cows that an induced hyperketonemia decreased plasma glucose and glucagon concentration, and affected systemic as well as local mammary metabolism and the immune response of the mammary gland. The pioneering outcome was that the thought essentiality of glucose for the exclusively on this particular nutrient insisting immune system can be partially replaced by BHBA. Recently, we investigated the effects of BHBA infusions shortly before and after parturition on glucose and lipid metabolism of dairy cows. Whereas the effects of BHBA on glucose metabolism were independent of the lactational stage, in particular the responses of the lipid metabolism changed with the physiological stage relative to parturition. Interestingly, despite elevated BHBA and NEFA concentrations postpartum, a further elevation of BHBA concentrations caused a decrease of plasma NEFA. In early lactation, the main portion of hepatic glucose output is used for lactose production for milk synthesis in the mammary gland. However, alternative energy sources are required for the metabolism of peripheral tissues including the immune system. At the onset of lactation, NEFA are excessively mobilized beyond the actual requirements. Enhancing the NEB by omitting concentrate supplementation in the second week of lactation, however, did not result in an elevated metabolic load compared to adequately fed cows. When providing glucose directly via infusion in late gestation and early lactation, feed intake decreased, while milk yield increased. The concomitant insulin resistance in early lactation furthermore forces a directed nutrient supply for the mammary gland, but not for other tissues. Though metabolic load in early lactation is known to be associated with an increased risk of production diseases, in a long-term field study we could not identify a causal link to longevity. In conclusion, glucose, NEFA and BHBA represent energy and nutrient sources with innate characteristics affecting the success of adaptation to lactation.

Effects of hyperketonemia within the first six weeks of lactation on milk production and fertility

J. Ruoff, S. Borchardt, A. Mahrt and W. Heuwieser
Clinic for animal reproduction, Veterinary Medicine, Königsweg 65 Haus 27, 14163 Berlin, Germany; julia.ruoff@fu-berlin.de

The first 2 weeks after calving have been described as the main risk period for hyperketonemia (HYK). However, it was recently shown that dairy cows continued to be at risk for HYK until at least 42 DIM. The objectives of our study were to describe the occurence of hyperketonemia (HYK) within the first six weeks of lactation and to evaluate the effects of HYK on milk production, reproductive performance and early lactation culling risk. A total of 655 dairy cows from 6 commercial dairy farms in Germany were enrolled between 1 and 4 DIM. Cows were tested twice weekly using an electronic handheld meter for β-hydroxybutyrate (BHBA) for an examination period of 42 days resulting in 12 test results per cow. Hyperketonemia was defined as a BHBA concentration ≥ 1.2 mmol/l. The onset of HYK was described as early onset (first HYK event within the first 2 weeks) and late onset (first HYK event in week 3 to 6 postpartum). The effects of onset of HYK within the first six weeks of lactation on milk production (1st test day milk yield and 100 DIM milk yield), reproductive performance (time to first service, first service conception risk and pregnancy risk within 200 DIM) and on early lactation culling risk were analyzed using a generalized linear mixed model. Cumulative incidence of HYK was 48% and 72% for primiparous and multiparous cows, respectively. Peak incidence was in week 1.0 for primiparous cows and in week 2.5 for multiparous cows. Mean prevalence was 17.5%. In total, 72% of HYK positive cows had a negative test result 3 to 4 days later after the initial diagnosis of HYK. Cows with early onset of HYK had a higher 1st test day milk yield (+3.0 kg/d, $P<0.001$) and 100 DIM milk production (+301.6 kg; $P<0.001$) compared to non-ketotic cows. There was no effect of late onset of ketosis on 1st test day milk yield and 100 DIM milk production. There were no effects of HYK on the time to first service, first service conception risk and pregnancy risk within 200 DIM, irrespective of onset of ketosis and no effect on culling risk. In total, 72% of HYK positive cows had a negative test result after the initial diagnosis of HYK which should be considered at future treatment studies. Cows with early onset of HYK had a higher milk production compared to non-ketotic cows. HYK was not associated with negative effects on reproduction and early lactation culling risk. HYK in early lactation seems to be part of a physiological adaptational response to negative energy balance in transition dairy cows.

Diurnal differences in milk composition and their influence on *in vitro* growth of *S. aureus*

S.W.F. Eisenberg[1], E.M. Boerhout[2], L. Ravesloot[1], A.J.J.M. Daemen[1], L. Benedictus[1], V.P.M.G. Rutten[1,3] and A.P. Koets[1,4]
[1]Faculty of Veterinary Medicine, Yalelaan, 3584CL Utrecht, the Netherlands, [2]MSD Animal Health, Wim de Körverstraat, 5830 AA Boxmeer, the Netherlands, [3]Faculty of Veterinary Science, Private Bag X04, Onderstepoort 0110, South Africa, [4]Central Veterinary Institute, Edelhertweg 15, 8200 AB Lelystad, the Netherlands; eveline.boerhout@merck.com

In experimental intramammary inoculation studies it has been observed that mastitis susceptibility is influenced amongst others by cow factors such as age, lactation stage and teat and udder anatomy as well as somatic cell count. As mastitis susceptibility also differs between quarters of a cow, differences in milk composition between quarters might play a role. To identify milk characteristics associated with these differences, quarter milk samples of morning and evening milk were collected and analysed extensively for their composition i.c. protein, fat, lactose, urea, lactoferrin, lactoperoxidase, and β-lactoglobulin concentrations, somatic cell count (SCC), and antibodies against *Staphylococcus aureus* (SA). Furthermore, *in vitro* growth of SA in fresh quarter milk samples was determined. A mixed model analysis was performed to identify associations between growth of SA and milk composition. All measured parameters differed significantly between quarters and also between morning and evening milk with the exception of lactose levels. In addition, quantitative growth of SA was significantly different in morning milk compared to evening milk. Mixed model analysis revealed that replication of SA was negatively associated with the presence of fat (1% increase reduced colony forming unit count by 42%), SA specific IgG1 antibodies (a 1 log2 increase of SA specific antibodies decreased cfu count by 26%), bacterial contamination of the milk sample (sterile milk increased cfu count by 74%) and morning milk (in morning milk cfu count was reduced by 71% compared to evening milk). Data presented here confirm earlier studies which describe an inhibitory effect of other bacteria on SA replication. The significant time effect supports the theory that milk changes influence SA growth. Although all determined milk components differed significantly between quarters no significant association with SA replication was identified with the exception of fat and IgG1. The bactericidal effect of fat was assumed to occur due to activation of lipolysis by milk handling and can most likely be neglected for *in vivo* relevance. The fact that SA specific IgG1 titers were negatively associated with SA growth encourages the ongoing efforts to develop a vaccine against SA induced mastitis.

The effect of dry period length and concentrate level on metabolic health in dairy cows

R.J. Van Hoeij[1], J. Dijkstra[2], R.M. Bruckmaier[3], J.J. Gross[3], T.J.G.M. Lam[4], B. Kemp[1] and A.T.M. Van Knegsel[1]
[1]*Wageningen University, Animal Sciences, Adaptation Physiology Group, P.O. Box 338, 6700 AH, Wageningen, the Netherlands,* [2]*Wageningen University, Animal Sciences, Animal Nutrition Group, P.O. Box 338, 6700 AH, Wageningen, the Netherlands,* [3]*University of Bern, Veterinary Physiology, Vetsuisse Faculty, Bremgartenstrasse 109a, 3001 Bern, Switzerland,* [4]*Utrecht University, Department Farm Animal Health, P.O. Box 80151, 3508 TD, Utrecht, the Netherlands; renny.vanhoeij@wur.nl*

Cows without a dry period (0-d DP) have a better energy balance (EB) than cows with a short dry period (30-d), due to reduced milk production in the subsequent lactation. Lower milk production results in lower energy demands, and potentially requires less energy intake. Lower energy intake, through reduction of concentrates offered, reduces feed costs and is potentially beneficial for net herd returns and environmental impact of the herd. It is unclear if feeding less energy results in even lower milk production or a decreased EB in early lactation. The aim of this study was to analyse the effect of a 0-d DP, with a 84% or 100% level of concentrates or a 30-d DP with a 100% level of concentrates on energy balance and plasma metabolites between week -4 and week 7 relative to calving. Holstein-Friesian dairy cows (n=127) were randomly assigned to three groups with two DP lengths (0 or 30 days). Cows with a 0-d DP were fed either 84% (0-d DP-C84%) or 100% (0-d DP-C100%) of the concentrate level of cows with a 30-d DP (30-d DP-C100%). Postpartum milk yield, FPCM yield, and yield of lactose, fat, and protein were greater in cows with a 30-d DP-C100%, than in cows with a 0-d DP-C84% or 0-d DP-C100% ($P<0.05$). Dry matter intake, basal ration intake, and plasma glucose concentration were greater in cows with a 0-d DP-C84% or a 0-d DP-C100%, compared with cows with a 30-d DP-C100% ($P<0.05$). Concentrate intake was lower in cows with a 0-d DP-C84%, than in cows with a 0-d DP-C100% or a 30-d DP-C100% ($P<0.01$). The EB was lower and plasma NEFA and BHBA concentration was higher in cows with a 30-d DP-C100%, than in cows with a 0-d DP-C84% or a 0-d DP-C100% ($P<0.01$). Lower concentrate intake in cows with a 0-d DP and C84% led to a greater intake of basal ration but a non-significant 5% lower NE$_L$ intake, than in cows with a 0-d DP and C100%. Partial compensation of concentrate intake with basal ration shows that cows with a 0-d DP can consume sufficient energy for milk production through basal ration, without detrimental effects on EB. Feeding a reduced level of concentrates after a 0-d DP can be beneficial for roughage intake and rumination, and may be relevant for prevention of subacute ruminal acidosis in early lactation. Studies are ongoing to evaluate the effects of dietary energy availability and DP length on lactation.

Estimation of heritability and repeatability for milk fever in Costa Rican dairy cattle

A. Saborío-Montero[1], B. Vargas-Leitón[2], J.J. Romero-Zúñiga[2] and J. Camacho[2]
[1]University of Costa Rica, Animal Science Department and Animal Nutrition Research Center, San José, 11501 San Pedro, Montes de Oca, Costa Rica, [2]National University of Costa Rica, Population Medicine Research Program, Veterinary Medicine School, Heredia, 40701, Lagunilla, Costa Rica; alesabor@gmail.com

The aim of this study was to estimate genetic parameters and perform genetic evaluation for milk fever in Costa Rican dairy cattle. A farm-based management information system (VAMPP) was used to collect 211 956 lactation records, from 61,611 cows, 2 breeds (Holstein and Jersey) and 125 herds. The pedigree file comprised 70,834 animals born between years 1989 and 2013 and distributed across 16 generations. Data was analyzed using an animal model with repeatability. The model included breed, herd, parity, month/year of calving as fixed effects, and cow additive genetic, permanent environmental and herd×sire interaction as random effects. The model was fit using a Generalized Linear Mixed Models (GLMM) approach, as implemented in ASReml 4.0™ software, assuming two different distributions for milk fever events: Normal (linear model) and Binomial (threshold model). A total of 4,097 (1.93%) clinical cases of milk fever were reported within this population. For the linear model, heritability and repeatability were, respectively, 0.01 (SE=0.002) and 0.03 (SE=0.002). For the threshold model, the variance component for permanent environmental effect was fixed to cero by the optimization algorithm, which resulted in an equal value of 0.11 (SE=0.012) for heritability and repeatability. The correlation between BLUPs of both models was 0.90. The accuracy of the estimated BLUPs were 0.33 (SD=0.12) for the linear model and 0.25 (SD=0.14) for the threshold model. Heritability for milk fever within this population is low, though significant. Estimates of variance components for random effects were more stable with the linear compared to the threshold model.

Relationship between metabolism and natural autoantibodies in dairy cows with different dry period length

N. Mayasari[1,2], J. Chen[2], G. De Vries Reilingh[2], J.J. Gross[3], R.M. Bruckmaier[3], B. Kemp[2], H.K. Parmentier[2] and A.T.M. Van Knegsel[2]
[1]Universitas Padjadjaran, Faculty of Animal Husbandry, Jalan Raya Bandung Sumedang Km. 21, 45363, Jatinangor, Indonesia, [2]Wageningen University, Adaptation Physiology Group, Department of Animal Science, P.O. Box 338, 6700 AH Wageningen, the Netherlands, [3]University of Bern, Veterinary Physiology, Vetsuisse Faculty, Bremgartenstrasse 109a, 3012 Bern, Switzerland; novi.mayasari@wur.nl

Natural autoantibodies (NAAb) maintain homeostasis and may prevent infections. The objective of this study was to evaluate the effects of dry period length (0-, 30-, or 60-d) and dietary energy source on levels of NAAb in plasma binding glutamate dehydrogenase (GD) and carbonic anhydrase (CA). In total, 167 Holstein-Friesian dairy cows were randomly assigned to treatments. Treatments consisted of 3 dry period lengths: 0-, 30- or 60-d, and 2 early lactation diets (glucogenic or lipogenic), resulting in a 3×2 factorial design. Blood was sampled weekly from week -3 until 9 relative to calving. Liver samples were collected in week -2, 2, and 4 relative to calving. Feed intake and milk yield was determined daily and pooled per week. Energy balance was calculated per week. Cows with a 30-d dry period had increased levels of IgM binding CA in plasma compared with cows with a 60-d dry period. Cows with a 0-d dry period had no difference on titers of IgM binding CA compared with cows with a 30-d or 60-d dry period. From week -3 until 9 relative to calving, levels of IgM binding CA tended to have a positive relationship with energy balance. Moreover, levels of IgM binding CA were positively related with non-esterified fatty acids concentration in plasma. Levels of IgG binding CA tended to have a positive relationship with insulin-like growth factor-I in plasma. Levels of both IgG and IgM binding GD were positively related with insulin concentration in plasma. The results of this study suggest that cows with a 30-d dry period not only had an improved energy balance but also had increased plasma titers of IgM binding CA compared with cows with a 60-d dry period. It is concluded that IgM binding CA in plasma might be an indicator for energy balance in dairy cows. Moreover, levels of IgG and IgM binding GD in plasma were associated with the metabolic hormone insulin. It is hypothesized that plasma NAAb levels may reflect metabolic status in dairy cows.

Effects of dry period length on lactation curve characteristics over 2 consecutive years

J. Chen[1], A. Kok[1,2], G.J. Remmelink[3], B. Kemp[1] and A.T.M. Van Knegsel[1]
[1]Wageningen University, Adaptation Physiology Group, Department of Animal Sciences, P.O. Box 338, 6700 AH Wageningen, the Netherlands, [2]Wageningen University, Animal Production Systems Group, Department of Animal Sciences, P.O. Box 338, 6700 AH Wageningen, the Netherlands, [3]Wageningen University and Research Centre, Livestock Research, P.O. Box 338, 6700 AH Wageningen, the Netherlands; juncai.chen@wur.nl

In recent years, interest in shortening the dry period for dairy cows has increased. Shortening and omitting the dry period improves energy balance, metabolic health, and fertility, but reduces milk yield after calving. The effects of dry period length on lactation curve characteristics were still unclear. Therefore, the objective of this study was to evaluate the effects of dry period length on lactation curve characteristics over 2 consecutive years. Holstein-Friesian dairy cows (n=167) were assigned randomly to 1 of 3 dry period lengths (0-, 30-, or 60-d). Cows had the same dry period for 2 consecutive years. Fat- and protein-corrected milk (FPCM) was recorded weekly. A Wilmink lactation curve was modeled for FPCM yield for each lactation. The cumulative 305-d FPCM yield (FPCM 305) was calculated by summing the estimated daily FPCM yield until 305 DIM. The 365-d FPCM yield (FPCM365) was calculated by summing FPCM305 and FPCM produced in the 60 d pre-calving. The lactation persistency was defined as daily reduction in estimated FPCM yield (kg/d) from 100 DIM to 280 DIM. In the first year, cows with a 0- or 30-d dry period had lower FPCM305, lower peak yield, and later peak time compared with cows with a 60-d dry period ($P<0.01$). Cows with a 30-d dry period had similar FPCM365 compared with cows with a 60-d dry period in the first year. Young cows (parity = 2) with a 0-d dry period had a greater reduction in FPCM305 and peak yield compared with older cows (parity >2) with a 0-d dry period. In the second year, cows with a 0- or 30-d dry period had lower peak yield ($P<0.01$) and cows with a 0-d dry period tended to have lower FPCM305 ($P=0.09$) compared with cows with a 60-d dry period. No effects of dry period length on FPCM365 were found in the second year. In both years, shortening or omitting dry period had no effect on lactation persistency. In conclusion, shortening or omitting the dry period resulted in lower peak yield, later peak time, and lower FPCM305, and the effects were more pronounced in the first year after implementation of dry period length treatment and in young cows compared with the second year and older cows, respectively. Moreover, the additional FPCM produced pre-calving in cows with a 0- or 30-d dry period could compensate FPCM305 losses in the subsequent lactation, especially in the second year.

Alterations of circulating NEFA, BHBA and lipid profile following intravenous glucose administration

M. Pourjafar, K. Badiei, A. Chalmeh, M. Mohamadi and F. Momenifar
School of Veterinary Medicine, Shiraz University, School of Veterinary Medicine, Department of Clinical Studies, 7144169155, Iran; pourjafarmehrdad@yahoo.com

Providing energy demands with emphasis on glucose supply can prevent metabolic disorders in high producing dairy cows. Hence, we hypothesized that bolus intravenous glucose administration may change the concentrations of circulating NEFA, BHBA and lipid profile to prevent and control metabolic dysfunctions in dairy cows. This research was carried out at winter 2014 on 25 multiparous Holstein dairy cows. Milk production was about 10,000 kg for year, an average of 3.6 of milk fat %, and 3.3 of milk protein %. All the animals were clinically healthy and body condition score (BCS) was estimated based on 0 to 5 system. Cattle were divided into 5 equal groups comprising early, mid and late lactations, far-off and close-up dry periods. Blood sample was taken immediately after catheterization, and dextrose 50% was administered at 500 mg/kg, 10 ml/kg/h, subsequently. Blood samples were collected from all cows through the fixed catheter prior to and 1, 2, 3 and 4 h after dextrose 50% infusion in plain tubes. After sera separation, β-hydroxy butyric acid (BHBA), non-esterified fatty acid (NEFA), triglyceride, cholesterol, high, low and very low density lipoproteins were detected in all samples. Serum concentrations of NEFA and BHBA in early and mid lactation cows were significantly higher than late lactation animals ($P<0.05$). Serum concentrations of NEFA and BHBA in close up dry cows were significantly higher than far off dry ones ($P<0.05$). Baseline levels of cholesterol in mid and late lactation were significantly higher than other groups. The level of low density lipoprotein in mid lactation cows was higher than others, significantly. The results of this study demonstrated that bolus intravenous glucose infusion can influence metabolism in high producing Holstein dairy cows. The changing patterns of circulating metabolic profile indicated that glucose is an important direct controller of metabolic interactions and responses in dairy cows in various production states. It could be concluded that high energy demands for lactogenesis, gravid uterus and negative energy balance are the main reasons for metabolic disorders of high producing Holstein dairy cows.

Performance and long-chain fatty acids in milk and blood of dairy cows fed a corn silage-based diet

C. Weber[1], A. Tröscher[2], A. Starke[3], H. Kienberger[4], M. Rychlik[4] and H.M. Hammon[1]
[1]Leibniz Institute for Farm Animal Biology (FBN), Wilhelm-Stahl-Allee 2, 18196 Dummerstorf, Germany, [2]BASF, Limburgerhof, 68623 Lampertheim, Germany, [3]University of Leipzig, An den Tierkliniken 11, 04103 Leipzig, Germany, [4]Technical University of Munich, Alte Akademie 10, 85354 Freising, Germany; hammon@fbn-dummerstorf.de

Diets fed to dairy cows contain primarily corn silage but less grass silage, providing minor amounts of essential fatty acids (EFA), particularly alpha-linolenic acid (ALA). Feeding a diet with reduced fat and ALA content results in an impaired ALA availability and in less rumen production of conjugated linoleic acid (CLA), thus leading to lower CLA availability, too. To verify these assumptions, we fed a total mixed ration (TMR) based on corn silage with a low fat content to provoke a reduced dietary fat and ALA supply. We studied performance and fatty acids in milk and blood plasma lipid fractions in five lactating cows (57 DIM ± 12 d at start of the study), that were investigated for 24 wk after changing from a grass/corn silage based TMR (GS) to a solely corn silage based TMR (CS). Diets were similar in energy and protein content (6.8 MJ NEL/kg of dry matter (DM), crude protein 155 g/kg DM). Crude fat was lower in CS than in GS (20.38 vs 30.99 g/kg DM). Content of linoleic acid (LA) was quite similar (10.8 and 11.7 g/kg DM in CS and GS), but ALA content was much lower in CS than in GS diet (1.0 vs 6.2 g/kg DM). Dry matter intake (DMI), milk yield and milk composition were measured weekly. Fatty acid composition in milk was measured in wk -1, 2, 4, 6, 8, 16, 20, 24, and in plasma in wk -1, 8, 16, 24 relative to diet change. Data were analysed by mixed model of SAS with time as fixed effect. Energy intake and DMI increased, but total fat intake decreased with CS diet ($P<0.001$). Intake of LA increased with time but ALA intake dropped down with the CS diet ($P<0.001$). Milk yield, energy-corrected milk and fat and protein yield declined with time ($P<0.001$), but protein and fat content in milk increased at the same time ($P<0.01$). Concentration of ALA and its relative amount in milk fat decreased ($P<0.001$), whereas relative amount of LA in milk fat increased ($P<0.001$), but LA concentration in milk was unaltered. Concentration of c9, t11 CLA and t11 vaccenic acid decreased ($P<0.001$) in milk and in milk fat with CS feeding. ALA concentration and its relative amount decreased after CS feeding ($P<0.001$) in the free fatty acid, the neutral lipid and the phospholipid fraction. At the same time, relative amount of LA increased in the neutral lipid fraction and concentration of LA decreased in the free fatty acid fraction ($P<0.001$). Our results show that the CS diet reduces ALA content in milk fat and plasma lipid fractions and results in a reduced ALA status in dairy cows.

Adipose tissue INSR and GLUT4 expression with reference to body condition score in Holstein cows

H. Jaakson[1], P. Karis[1], K. Ling[1], J. Samarütel[1], A. Ilves[1], E. Reimann[1], P. Pärn[1], R. Bruckmaier[2], J. Gross[2] and M. Ots[1]
[1]*Estonian University of Life Sciences, Kreutzwaldi 46, 51006 Tartu, Estonia,* [2]*University of Bern, Bremgartenstr. 109a, 3001 Bern, Switzerland; priit.karis@student.emu.ee*

Glucose uptake in adipose tissue is mediated by binding of insulin with its receptor (INSR) leading to the expression of insulin-dependent glucose transporters 4 (GLUT4). At the beginning of lactation insulin resistance develops that is presumably linked to reduced number and affinity of INSR as well as to altered post-receptor signalling that leads to supressed expression of GLUT4. Aim of the present study was to examine the effect of body condition score (BCS) during dry period on the expression of mRNA and protein of INSR and GLUT4 in the adipose tissue of Holstein cows three weeks pre- (w-3) and postpartum (w3). Cows (n=42) were divided according to BCS four weeks prepartum into three groups: BCS≤3.0 (Thin, T); BCS=3.25-3.5 (Optimal, O); BCS≥3.75 (Fat, F). Biopsies were taken from pin bone region in w-3 and w3; mRNAs abundance was measured with real-time PCR; proteins were quantified with ELISA. Student's T-test was used to analyse differences; significance was declared at $P<0.05$. In w-3 INSR mRNA abundance was lower in all groups followed by about 6-fold ($P<0.05$), 5-fold ($P<0.01$) and 3-fold ($P<0.01$) increase to w3 in T, O and F groups respectively. In w3 the highest INSR mRNA level was observed in T group, differing from the lowest level F group ($P<0.05$). INSR protein expression did not follow the pattern of its mRNA: in w-3 the highest protein level was measured in T and the lowest in O group ($P<0.05$); in all groups following changes as well as differences in w3 were not significant. The pattern of GLUT4 mRNA abundance was similar to INSR protein. GLUT4 protein level in w-3 was highest in O and lowest in F group ($P<0.05$). About 2-fold decrease from w-3 to w3 in T and O groups ($P<0.001$), along with largely unchanged level in F group, resulted in the highest protein level in F and lowest in T group ($P<0.05$). Our results reveal that there are no explicit relationships between mRNA and protein expression of INSR and GLUT4. Despite the several-fold increase of INSR mRNA postpartum and therefore the increased potential for INSR protein synthesis the protein levels stayed the same as prepartum; furthermore, regardless of the almost unchanged expression of INSR protein and GLUT4 mRNA there was noticeable decrease of GLUT4 protein levels in T and O groups postpartum. Our results suggest inhibition of INSR and GLUT4 expression at post-transcriptional level and support the statement about insulin resistance manifestation at post-receptor level. This study was supported by institutional research funding (IUT 8-1) of the Estonian Ministry of Education and Research.

Season of birth affects 305 d milk and fat yield during first lactation in HF heifers

M. Van Eetvelde[1], M. Pierre[1], L. Vandaele[2] and G. Opsomer[1]
[1]Ghent University, Department of Reproduction, Obstetrics and Herd health, Salisburylaan 133, 9820 Merelbeke, Belgium, [2]Institute for Agricultural and Fisheries Research, Scheldeweg 68, 9090 Melle, Belgium; geert.opsomer@ugent.be

In cattle, as in several other species, both the pre- and early postnatal environment are known to have long-term consequences on the health and production of the offspring. The aim of the present study was to assess environmental (season of birth and calving) and offspring (weight and gender) effects on the milk yield during first lactation in Holstein Friesian (HF) heifers. Seventy-nine female HF calves were followed from birth until second parturition in 3 herds in Flanders (Belgium). Body weight was collected at birth and first parturition, as well as gender and birth weight of their offspring. Season of birth and calving were grouped as follows: Winter (21 December to 20 March), Spring (21 March to 20 June), Summer (21 June to 20 September) and Fall (21 September to 20 December). After second parturition, 305 days milk as well as fat and protein yields of the first lactation were calculated based on monthly milk recordings. Linear mixed models, with herd as a random factor, were built to assess the factors influencing first lactation yield and results are presented as LSMeans. Most heifers were born during Fall (44%) and Spring (24%), with only 17% and 15% of heifers born in Winter and Summer, respectively. Heifers calved at an age of 24.7±2.02 months, weighing on average 643±61.0 kg. At first parturition, 40 female and 39 male calves were born with an average birth weight of 40.3±50.56 kg, while in the subsequent lactation, heifers produced a 305 d milk yield of 8,348±1,230.4 kg, with 4.2±0.47% fat and 3.5±0.21% protein. Weight at calving had a significant effect on the first lactation 305 d milk yield, with heavier heifers producing more milk ($P=0.002$). Milk yield was also affected by season of birth, with the lowest production in heifers born in Winter (7,818±677.3 kg) and a significantly higher production in heifers born in Fall (8,745±634.5 kg; $P=0.04$). Despite the fact that the season of birth and calving was identical for most (65%) of the heifers, calving season did not have a significant effect on milk yield. Finally, heifers born in Summer produced milk with a fat content of 4.4±0.19%, compared to only 4.0±0.15% in heifers born in Fall ($P=0.04$). Results of the study suggest season of birth rather than season of calving to influence first lactation milk and fat yield in HF heifers. As milk yield was lowest in heifers born during colder and darker days while highest in heifers born during longer and hotter days, the effect of birth season might be attributed to differences in temperature or photoperiod at the end of their term in utero.

Impact of 25-hydroxyvitamin D3 combined with an acidifying diet on dairy cows' calcium homeostasis

I. Cohrs[1], M.R. Wilkens[2], E. Azem[3], B. Schröder[2] and G. Breves[2]
[1]University of Veterinary Medicine Hannover Foundation, Clinic for Cattle, Bischofsholer Damm 15, 30173 Hannover, Germany, [2]University of Veterinary Medicine Hannover Foundation, Department of Physiology, Bischofsholer Damm 15, 30173 Hannover, Germany, [3]DSM Nutritional Products, P.O. Box 2676, 4002 Basel, Switzerland; imkecohrs@gmx.de

A previous, preliminary study has shown an age-dependent beneficial effect of an oral supplementation with 25-hydroxyvitamin D_3 (25-OHD_3) on peripartal calcium (Ca) plasma concentrations of cows kept on an acidifying diet. Therefore, two different dosages of 25-OHD_3 were tested once again with special emphasis on duration of treatment and lactation number. Starting on 270th day of gestation 90 cows entering at least 2nd lactation with the following parturition were divided into three groups: control, 4 mg 25-OHD_3 and 6 mg 25-OHD_3. Due to variable lengths of gestation, cows had to be assigned to groups of short and long duration of treatment in retrospect. Animals were sampled every other day until parturition, 0, 6, 12, 24 and 48 h after parturition (p.p.) and on day 4 p.p. Plasma concentrations of Ca, 25-OHD_3, calcitriol, parathyroid hormone (PTH) and CrossLaps (CL) as a bone resorption marker were analyzed and evaluated by using a 3-way ANOVA for repeated measurements with the factors dosage (0, 4, 6 mg/day), lactation number (2nd vs ≥3rd) and duration of treatment (3-10 vs 11-16 days). Plasma concentrations of 25-OHD_3 were increased by the supplementation during the treatment period from the 270th day of gestation until parturition as a function of duration of treatment and dosage. Influence of parity led to significantly higher peripartal (0-24 h p.p.) plasma concentrations of PTH and calcitriol in cows entering ≥3rd lactation, but had no effect on CL. The lowest CL plasma concentrations were detected in cows fed 6 mg 25-OHD_3 for 11-16 days. At parturition Ca plasma concentrations decreased in all cows. Supplementation did not affect Ca plasma concentrations in cows entering 2nd lactation, but led to significantly higher Ca plasma concentrations before parturition and a steeper increase afterwards in response to long treatment with 6 mg 25-OHD_3 in older cows. The lowest Ca plasma concentrations at parturition were observed for long treatment with 4 mg 25-OHD_3. From the observed changes in plasma concentrations of CL and Ca it may be concluded that daily supplementation of 6 mg 25-OHD_3 combined with anionic salts leads to an enhanced gastrointestinal absorption of Ca from the diet, an increased storage of Ca in bone and a faster release of Ca at the onset of lactation. However, these effects depend on respective increases in plasma concentrations of 25-OHD_3 and age of the animals.

Effects of cinnamon supplementation on performance and metabolic responses of transition dairy cows

H. Vakili[1], A.R. Alizadeh[1,2], A. Ghorbani[1], R.M. Bruckmaier[3], H. Sauerwein[2] and H. Sadri[2]
[1]Department of Animal Science, Saveh Branch, Islamic Azad University, Saveh, Iran, [2]Institute of Animal Science, Physiology & Hygiene Unit, University of Bonn, Bonn, Germany, [3]Veterinary Physiology, Vetsuisse Faculty, University of Bern, Bern, Switzerland; hsadri@uni-bonn.de

For dairy cows, impaired insulin regulation of energy metabolism is considered as etiologic key component for metabolic diseases typically occurring during the transition from pregnancy to lactation. There is evidence that cinnamon (CIN) exhibits insulin-potentiating activity. In condideration that CIN supplementation may improve insulin sensitivity, we hypothesized that performance and metabolic responses of transition dairy cows will profit from CIN supplementation. Twenty four dry Holstein cows in late gestation were studied from 4 weeks before anticipated calving date until 4 weeks thereafter. Cows (n=8/treatment) were assigned to either the control group (CTR; without supplementation) or the supplementation groups [supplemental CIN at 20 (LCIN) or 40 (HCIN) g/cow/day]. Blood samples were collected on d -21, -7, 1, 2, 7, 14, and 21 relative to calving. The serum concentrations of insulin, non-esterified fatty acids (NEFA), glucose, and beta-hydroxybutyrate (BHBA) were measured and an index estimating insulin sensitivity (RQUICKI) was calculated from the former 3 variables. Data were analyzed by the MIXED model with treatment, time, and interaction of treatment and time as the fixed effects and cow as the random effect. There was no CIN effect on prepartum dry matter intake or postpartum milk yield and composition. The serum concentrations of glucose and insulin did not differ among the groups, but changed over time ($P<0.001$) and followed a similar pattern in all groups. No treatment by time interaction was observed for the serum concentrations of glucose and insulin. The serum NEFA concentrations were affected by treatment, time, and interaction between treatment and time ($P≤0.04$). The serum NEFA concentrations were greater ($P<0.05$) on d 2, 7, and 14 in LCIN than in CTR. The serum concentrations of BHBA were affected by CIN supplementation and time ($P≤0.008$). On d 14, and 21, cows in the supplementation groups had greater ($P<0.05$) serum BHBA concentrations than the cows in the CTR group. RQUICKI did not differ among the treatments, but changed over time ($P=0.03$). In conclusion, prepartum DMI and lactation performance of dairy cows were not affected by the dietary CIN. The data suggests lipolytic and ketogenic effects of CIN supplementation in periparturient dairy cows at the dosage used, as indicated by the increased concentrations of NEFA and BHBA post partum.

Predicting postpartum disorders with prepartum metabolic markers in dairy cows

S.G.A. Van Der Drift, I.M.G.A. Santman-Berends and G.H.M. Counotte
Gezondheidsdienst voor Dieren, R&D, P.O. Box 9, 7400 AA Deventer, the Netherlands;
s.v.d.drift@gddiergezondheid.nl

Management and feeding practices during the dry period have a direct impact on the health of cows in the periparturient period. Recent literature suggests that metabolic indicators in dry cows can be used to predict the risk for postpartum disorders. The objective of the study was to assess the association between prepartum serum NEFA, BHBA, haptoglobin and urea concentrations relative to the incidence of postpartum disorders in dairy cows. Between September 2014 and April 2015, serum samples of 625 dry cows from 40 Dutch dairy herds were collected and analysed for NEFA, BHBA, haptoglobin, urea, and albumin. Postpartum disorders occurring between parturition and 100 DIM were registered. Observations with missing calving dates or from cows that were not sampled between 60 days prepartum and parturition (during the dry cow period) were removed from the dataset. The final dataset contained observations from 551 cows. Multivariate logistic regression models were used to predict high or low risk for development of specific postpartum disorders based on the information of the metabolic markers. A random herd effect was included to control for the effect of clustering of observations within herds. Cross-validation techniques without the inclusion of the random herd effect were used to evaluate the models. Serum concentrations of NEFA and BHBA increased and urea and albumin concentrations decreased in cows with decreasing time to parturition at moment of sampling ($P<0.01$ for all three markers). A total of 28.2% of cows developed a postpartum disorder. Best predictive models were obtained for the disorders retentio secundinarum (prevalence 2.3%) and endometritis (prevalence 6.3%). The model for retentio secundinarum included serum haptoglobin and NEFA concentrations within 30 days before calving. With every increase in the serum haptoglobin concentration of 1 g/l, cows had a significant higher odds (OR: 4.7 (CI 1.8-12.4)) for developing retentio secundinarum For serum NEFA concentrations, every increase of 1 mmol/l increased the OR for retentio secundinarum with 8.6 (CI 0.9-87.9). The model for endometritis included serum haptoglobin, BHBZ and urea concentrations within 30 days before calving. The OR for developing endometritis was 2.5 (CI 1.0-6.1) with every increase in the serum haptoglobin concentration of 1 g/l. The OR for developing endometritis was 2.3 (CI 0.8-6.7) and 17.1 (CI 4.3-67.8) for cows with BHBA concentrations between 0.55-0.90 and ≥0.90 mmol/l, respectively. Results from this study suggests that common metabolic indicators in dry cows could be used to predict the risk for postpartum disorders.

Changes in the serum BHB concentration before and after parturition in Iranian dairy cows

M. Sakha

Science and Research Branch, Islamic Azad University, Clinical Sciences, Faculty of Specialized Veterinary Sciences, Ashrafi Highway, Hesarak, 14515-755 Tehran, Iran; msakha@yahoo.com

Various tests are available for monitoring ketosis/subclinical ketosis in dairy herds. However, none of them has perfect sensitivity and specificity as compared with blood BHB. Therefore, measuring blood BHB concentration as the gold standard method is the most accurate test for herd monitoring. Serum BHB concentrations change in all group of cows throughout the entire lactation and the dry period. When sudden changes in diet are made or when food of different quality is substituted for a part of the ration, significant alterations in serum BHB concentration are to be expected. In cows with high concentrations of BHB (clinical ketosis), assessment of glucose concentrations may provide an useful additional indicator for the severity of the condition. Plasma glucose is of value in case of gross rather than marginal dietary deficits. The objective of this study were: (1) to characterize changes of BHB (along with glucose) concentrations in Iranian dairy cows; (2) to identify a cut-off point for BHB in the first weeks after calving; and (3) to correlate BHB and glucose concentrations during the dry and the lactation period. Blood samples were obtained from 13 Holstein cows(4-6 years old) 16, 8 and 1 week before calving and at 4 and 8 weeks after calving. The formulated diet was used for all cows. Daily milk yield was recorded and the number of lactations was also considered. The mean serum BHB concentrations (mmol/l) from the 5 consecutive sampling points were 0.58 ± 0.18, 0.58 ± 0.18, 0.78 ± 0.15, 1.04 ± 0.24, and 0.91 ± 0.11. The corresponding glucose concentrations (mg/dl) were 50.3 ± 7.91, 46.8 ± 5.44, 43.4 ± 3.90, 39.6 ± 3.40, and 42.1 ± 3.20. A significant increase in the BHB and a significant decrease in the glucose concentrations was observed one a month after parturition ($P<0.05$). There was a significant positive correlation between BHB concentration and age, milk production and parity ($P<0.01$). In conclusion, the concentration of BHB during lactation was greater than during the dry period, possibly due to the higher energy demand in lactating cows. BHB peaked one month after parturition in the sampling schedule applied herein. Based on the mean BHB concentration and the individual BHB values one month after parturition observed in this study, a reasonable cut-off point for BHB to detect subclinical ketosis in Iranian Holstein cows may be close to 1.2 mmol/l, however, further investigations are required to substantiate this threshold level.

Effects of 25-hydroxycholecalciferol on calcium balance and vitamin D metabolism in sheep

S. Klinger, G. Breves, B. Schröder and M.R. Wilkens
University of Veterinary Medicine Hannover, Foundation, Department of Physiology, Bischofsholer Damm 15/102, 30173 Hannover, Germany; mirja.wilkens@tiho-hannover.de

In a recent study on calcium (Ca) homeostasis of dairy cows during the transition period beneficial effects of the vitamin D metabolite 25-hydroxycholealciferol (25-OHD) in combination with a ration negative in dietary cation anion difference (DCAD) could be demonstrated. The aim of the present work was to attempt to identify the mechanisms of this 25-OHD effect. Ten female, non-lactating, non-pregnant sheep aged 12 months were divided into a placebo and a 25-OHD treated group. In a 1st series all animals were kept in metabolism crates for a control period of 6 days. During a 2nd series the sheep were fed a negative DCAD diet and treated daily with either a placebo or 0.6 µg 25-OHD per kg body weight. After the 2nd series the animals were sacrificed and renal as well as gastrointestinal tissue samples were taken to be analysed for gene products involved in Ca transport and vitamin D metabolism by qPCR. Daily renal Ca excretion was significantly enhanced with the diet negative in DCAD (0.05±0.01 vs 1.16±0.11 g). Interestingly, also apparent digestibility of Ca was significantly greater when the negative DCAD diet was fed compared to the control period (11.7±2.5 vs 19.0±1.9%). The additional supplementation with 25-OHD resulted in a further increase in apparent digestibility (26.1±1.8%). This observation obtained *in vivo* was in line with data on RNA quantification. In the jejunal mucosa expression of the apically located Ca channel TRPV6 and the basolateral plasma Ca-ATPase PMCA1b was significantly greater in the 25-OHD supplemented group. Furthermore, 25-OHD had an impact on vitamin D metabolism of the animals. The renal 1-α-hydroxylase, the enzyme that catalyses the transformation of 25-OHD to the biologically most active vitamin D metabolite 1,25-dihydroxycholealciferol, was significantly down-regulated by the treatment (to 15±4% of the expression determined in the control group). Additionally, a 20-fold up-regulation was found for the 24-hydroxylase, which inactivates several vitamin D metabolites. Taken together, a supplementation with 25-OHD can increase gastrointestinal Ca absorption and might therefore diminish the negative effects of a diet negative in DCAD on overall Ca balance. However, the observed impact on vitamin D metabolism has to be taken into consideration, especially when 25-OHD is used in animals experiencing rapid changes in Ca demand like dairy cows. This project was supported by the German Research Foundation (DFG WI 3668/1-1).

IGF-1 was not predictive for early post partum ketosis in a field study

V. Jacobs[1,2], M. Araujo[3], R. Tietze[1] and M. Schmicke[2]
[1]Veterinary Practice Dr. R. Tietze, Dorfstraße 31, 17209 Melz, Germany, [2]University of Veterinary Medicine, Clinic for Cattle, Endocrinology, Bischofsholer Damm 15, 30173 Hannover, Germany, [3]University of Zulia, Faculty of Veterinary Science, Maracaibo, Zulia 44011, Venezuela; marion.schmicke@tiho-hannover.de

We previously showed that the prepartum insulin-like growth factor-1 (IGF-1) concentration serve as indicator for post partum ketosis and was superior of NEFA measurement. However, in the preceded studies blood samples were taken from cows from one large scale dairy farm and all cows with ketosis (until three 3wks after calving) were included in statistical evacuations. The aim was to test, whether the IGF-1 concentration measured on day 263±3 after artificial insemination indicate specifically the cows at risk for clinical ketosis early post partum in cows from different farms. Secondly, it should be evaluated if cows suffering from clinical ketosis post partum (K-, n=6), clinical ketosis and any other production disease (K+; 0=6) and healthy controls (n=7) differ in their BHB, NEFA, growth hormone (GH), IGF-1 and insulin concentrations before and after standard ketosis treatment (dexamethasone, glucose and Catosal™). Therefore, cows at four farms were monitored with BHB measurements on the farms (d 3 and 8 after calving). If the BHB concentration was elevated, a blood sample was taken for laboratory BHB and NEFA measurement and a clinical examination was carried out. The cows with elevated BHB (>1.2 mmol/l) and clinical signs of ketosis were treated and additional blood samples were taken 1, 3 and 7 d after diagnose of ketosis. Seven healthy cows with low BHB values (>1.2 mmol/l) served as controls. In contrast to previous findings, the prepartal IGF-1 (ng/ml) concentration was comparable between healthy cows (190.7±36.2), K- (171.9±24.0) and K+ (170.4±64.0). The mean IGF-1 concentration on the different farms was comparable ($P>0.05$). The NEFA concentration (mmol/l) was higher in K+ (421.7±628.2) compared to K- (211.2±134.6) and healthy controls (132.7±31.2) before calving. However, after calving IGF-1 (ng/ml) and insulin (µU/ml) concentrations were higher in healthy cows (84.1±58; 14.7±5.7) compared to K- (52.9±35.2; 4.8±1.9) and K+ (32.0±0.1; 5.7±3.3). IGF-1 concentrations stayed constant after treatmnet of ketosis and were comparable between groups, whereas insulin increased and NEFA, BHB and GH decreased in K- and K+ ($P<0.05$). In conclusion, the IGF-1 concentration was numerically lower in cows developing a ketosis but seems questionable as risk parameter for ketosis in the field. After calving IGF-1 was lower in cows with severe ketosis and additional production disease corresponding to higher NEFA values in those cows. The Study was partly funded by the Schaumann Stiftung.

Optimization of dry cow management can influence natural antibody (Nab) levels in dairy cows

S. Carp-Van Dijken, I.M.G.A. Santman-Berends, G. Van Schaik, T.J.G.M. Lam and I.E.M. Den Uijl

Gezondheidsdienst voor Dieren, Afdeling Herkauwers, Postbus 9, 7400 AA Deventer, the Netherlands; s.v.dijken@gddiergezondheid.nl

Resilience plays an important role in the ability of cows to remain healthy. In previous research we found that natural antibody levels (IgM and IgG NAbs) combined with parity, SCC and postpartum disorders in the prior lactation could indicate whether a cow had a low or high risk for developing a disorder in the subsequent lactation. The aim of this study was to evaluate if postpartum disorders could be prevented by management optimisation and whether optimisation resulted in a change in NAb levels. In 29 Dutch dairy herds milk samples of cows were tested for NAb levels at each test-day milking from December 2013 to March 2015. From April 2014 on, for each study herd a plan was made to optimize dry cow management by a veterinarian specialized in feed in collaboration with the herd owners. During the optimisation which lasted until March 2015, the farmers were guided intensively. Test--day milk recording data, fertility records, identification and registration data and comprehensive data from disease registration systems were available. We evaluated whether the amount of postpartum disorders had changed during the period in which optimisation was conducted. A multilevel logistic regression model was used with postpartum disorder as dependent variable and period, parity, quality of optimisation and a random herd effect as independent variables. In addition, a linear regression model was used to evaluate the influence and quality of optimisation on NAb levels during the study period. Three measures for dry cows could be applied in all herds: 1. Improve daily dry matter intake 2. Optimisation of the ration 3. Stop with feeding leftover feed of the milking cows Other optimisation measures were often related to reduction of infectious pressure and reduction of stress. During the study period the percentage of postpartum disorders decreased from on average 21% prior to optimisation to 16% during optimisation. Higher NAb levels were known to be associated with higher incidence of postpartum disorders. It appeared that the NAb levels of the cows in the study herds decreased significantly in the period in which dry cow management was optimized. The decrease in NAb level was more evident in herds that applied the optimisation measures compared to herds that did not optimize their management. Our study showed that optimising dry cow management decreased Nab levels in dairy cows. Lower NAb levels contribute to a smaller proportion of cows defined as high risk for developing postpartum disease in the subsequent lactation and therefore the risk profile could be changed.

Experiment-corrected milk fat C18:1 cis-9 concentrations as energy status indicator in dairy cows

S. Jorjong[1], A.T.M. Van Knegsel[2], M. Hostens[3], F. Lannoo[1], G. Opsomer[3] and V. Fievez[1]
[1]Lanupro, Ghent University, Proefhoevestraat 10, 9090 Melle, Belgium, [2]Adaptation Physiology Group, Wageningen University, P.O. Box 338, 6700 AH Wageningen, the Netherlands, [3]Department of Reproduction, Obstetrics and Herd Health, Ghent University, Salisburylaan 133, 9820 Merelbeke, Belgium; sasitornj@gmail.com

Dairy cows in early lactation inevitably encounter a state of negative energy balance (NEB), reflected in elevated blood nonesterified fatty acids (NEFA). Released NEFA are partially transferred to the mammary gland and are particularly rich in C18:1 cis-9. A milk fat C18:1 cis-9 absolute cut-off value of 24 g/100 g fatty acids has been suggested as a promising biomarker of detrimental plasma NEFA ($\geq$0.6 mmol/l) in wk 2 of lactation. However, intra-experimental cross-validation of this absolute cut-off value performed poorly. Therefore, an experiment-corrected cut-off value has been proposed (4.11). The latter has been generated by subtracting an experiment-dependent basal level of milk fat C18:1 cis-9 from the original absolute cut-off value. This basal level was calculated as the average concentration of milk fat C18:1 cis-9 of cows with plasma NEFA concentrations below 0.6 mmol/l, which were considered 'healthy'. The current study assessed the potential of this experiment-corrected cut-off value of milk fat C18:1 cis-9 for prediction of NEB under practical circumstances, where information of NEFA concentrations is lacking. The experiment was conducted on a dairy farm with more than 2,000 cows. The dataset consisted of blood NEFA concentrations and milk fatty acid proportions. Primiparous (40) and multiparous (101) cows were sampled at 3 and 10 DIM. Milk samples were collected manually at the end of the morning milking. To simulate practical circumstances, the average milk fat C18:1 cis-9 concentration of the 65, 70, 75, 80, 85 or 90% lowest values were calculated and used as basal value. Average milk fat C18:1 cis-9 content of the 80% lowest values revealed most appropriate and corrected observations were calculated using the latter basal value. Validation of the formerly determined experiment-corrected cut-off value resulted in an overall accuracy between 75 and 80%. Higher sensitivities and odds ratio (OR) at d3 may indicate earlier sampling times to be of particular interest to rule out sick animals. The OR of 12 indicated cows with an experiment-corrected observation above 4.11 at d3 had 12 times more chance to reach blood NEFA concentrations above 0.6 mmol/l than the others. It was concluded that the experiment-dependent basal level could be calculated as the average of the 80% lowest milk fat C18:1 cis-9 concentrations in cows at the same lactation stage and under similar dietary conditions. The latter might impose problems on smaller farms, with only 5 to 10 calvings a month.

Colostrum composition assessment by on-farm tools at quarter and composite level in dairy cows

J.J. Gross, E.C. Kessler and R.M. Bruckmaier
Veterinary Physiology, Vetsuisse Faculty University of Bern, Bremgartenstrasse 109a, 3012 Bern, Switzerland; josef.gross@vetsuisse.unibe.ch

Control of colostrum quality is essential for successful calf rearing. Instruments for on-farm colostrum quality determination are widely used in dairy practice, but predominantly composite colostrum samples were considered so far, not taking potential variation between quarters into account. In cases of low composite colostrum quality, feeding of better quality colostrum from individual quarters might be beneficial. The objective of the present study was to identify relationships between colostrum color, colostrum quality assessed by a colostrometer and a Brix refractometer, and composition measured by different laboratory methods of colostrum at a quarter level. Quarter and composite colostrum samples from 17 primiparous and 11 multiparous Holstein cows were analyzed for total IgG, fat, protein and lactose content, and color was measured by a spectrophotometer. In the present study, an IgG concentration below 50 g/l as determined by ELISA was found in 14.3% of the analyzed quarter samples. Concentration and total mass of IgG in composite colostrum samples were higher in multiparous compared to primiparous cows. Specific gravity (SG) of colostrum of individual and composite samples was lower in primiparous compared to multiparous cows. Milk fat content was higher in quarter and composite colostrum samples of primiparous compared to multiparous dairy cows. Neither in primiparous nor in multiparous dairy cows clear relationships between IgG content and SG, Brix, and the color space coordinates L*, a*, and b* were detected. Interestingly, our results indicate that despite a similar range of the parameters investigated, correlations between those parameters can differ at quarter compared to composite level. Not only for SG and Brix determination, but also for the color space coordinates measured, correlation coefficients with IgG concentration of the respective samples were higher at a composite compared to the individual quarter level. In conclusion, accuracy and limitations of on-farm instruments estimating colostrum quality do also apply for quarter colostrum samples as they do for composite evaluations. Due to the variation of milk composition between individual quarters of a cow, correlation coefficients between colostral IgG concentration, SG, Brix-values, and colostrum color were in part poorer compared to composite samples.

Colostral immunoglobulin concentration is repeatable in consecutive lactations of dairy cows

J.J. Gross[1], G. Schüpbach-Regula[2] and R.M. Bruckmaier[1]
[1]*Veterinary Physiology, Vetsuisse Faculty University of Bern, Bremgartenstrasse 109a, 3012 Bern, Switzerland,* [2]*Veterinary Public Health Institute, Vetsuisse Faculty University of Bern, Schwarzenburgstrasse 155, 3097 Liebefeld, Switzerland; josef.gross@vetsuisse.unibe.ch*

Colostrum IgG concentration and yield vary tremendously among farms, cows, and between quarters within cows. The present study quantified changes in quarter colostrum characteristics up to three successive lactations. First colostrum was quarter collected within 4 h after parturition in the first 2 consecutive lactations from 12 cows, and colostrum was obtained from 14 multiparous dairy cows in 2, and 8 cows thereof in 3 consecutive lactations, respectively. Colostrum yield per quarter showed a high variation in both primiparous and multiparous dairy cows during consecutive lactations. Percentage distribution of colostrum yield between quarters within cows was similar from parity to parity. The differences in colostrum yield within the same quarter were higher in cows from first to second lactation compared to the differences within quarters of multiparous cows in consecutive lactations ($P<0.05$). The intra-class correlation coefficient (ICC) for quarter colostrum yield was found to be similar in cows from first to second parity (ICC=0.42) and within consecutive lactations of multiparous cows (ICC=0.44). Whereas position of the quarter did not influence colostrum yield in cows from first to second lactation, quarter colostrum yield in multiparous cows was higher in rear than in front quarters ($P<0.05$) with less changes in successive lactations. Concentration and mass of IgG in quarter-milked colostrum varied distinctly among quarters and cows in both primiparous and multiparous cows. In multiparous cows, higher values for quarter concentration and mass of IgG were observed when compared to primiparous cows, in particular in the rear quarters ($P<0.05$). Relative differences of IgG concentration and mass within quarters were higher in consecutive lactations of multiparous cows compared to differences within quarters of cows in the first two lactations ($P<0.05$). The ICC of colostral IgG concentration and mass within quarters of cows from first to second lactation was 0.52 and 0.67, respectively, and lower compared to the ICC of IgG concentration and mass within quarters during consecutive lactations of multiparous cows. In conclusion, IgG concentration and mass were shown to be more repeatable within quarters of multiparous compared to the first two lactations of dairy cows. Contrary, colostrum yield within quarters in consecutive lactations had only a moderate repeatability and seemed to be affected by factors other than genetics.

Metabolite profiles in blood and milk for cows with different dry period lengths in early lactation

W. Xu[1,2], A.T.M. Van Knegsel[2], D.B. De Koning[2], R. Van Hoeij[2], B. Kemp[2] and J.J.M. Vervoort[1]
[1]Wageningen University and Research centre, Laboratory of Biochemistry, Dreijenlaan 3, 6703 HA, the Netherlands, [2]Wageningen University and Research centre, Department of Animal Sciences, De Elst 1, 6708 WD Wageningen, the Netherlands; wei.xu@wur.nl

High-producing dairy cows experience a severe negative energy balance (NEB) during early lactation, with increased insulin resistance and body mobilization. The physiological status in NEB is associated with changed metabolite profiles in blood, and it can be expected that these changes also can be reflected in milk composition. However, there are only few reports about metabolite profiles in blood and milk for dairy cows in NEB. The objective of this study is to investigate metabolite profiles in plasma and milk of cows with different dry period (DP) lengths. Holstein-Friesian dairy cows (n=31, average daily milk production: 30.9 ± 1.6 kg/day; MEAN±SEM) were assigned randomly to one of two DP lengths (0 day or 30 days). Milk yield and feed intake were recorded daily and energy balance (EB) was determined weekly. Blood and milk were sampled every Thursday and Wednesday morning, respectively. Metabolite profiles in blood and milk were determined using 1H Nuclear Magnetic Resonance. Cows with a 0 day DP length had a higher EB (-144 ± 58 vs -365 ± 73 kJ/kg$^{0.75}$, $P<0.05$) and lower fat-and-protein-corrected-milk (27.8 ± 2.3 vs 34.2 ± 2.0 kg/d, $P<0.05$) compared with cows with a 30 days DP. Cows with a 0 day DP had lower plasma concentrations of hippurate, phenylalanine, tyrosine and creatinine ($P<0.05$) compared with cows with a 30 days DP. Moreover, higher amounts of choline and N-acetyl-sugar ($P<0.05$), and lower amounts of hippurate, ureum, fumaric acid, creatinine, glutamine, citrate, UDP-sugars and sugar-1-phosphates ($P<0.05$) were detected in milk of cows with a 0 day DP, compared with cows on a 30 days DP. In conclusion, results of this study indicate that cows with a 30 days DP have increased nitrogen and amino acid catabolism, possibly for increased DNA/RNA synthesis as ammonia from amino acid deamidation is needed for de novo nucleotide synthesis. The observation of an increase in sugar-1-phosphates in cows with a 30 days DP indicates that also more apoptosis is occurring. The increase in nitrogen metabolism and apoptosis indicates that both cell degradation and renewal occur at the same time in cows with a 30 days DP. Studies are ongoing to confirm these results in a larger dataset with extended metabolite and proteome datasets of both blood and milk samples.

Changing patterns of thyroid hormones following bolus intravenous glucose administration in sheep

K. Badiei, M. Pourjafar, A. Chalmeh, A. Mirzaei, M.H. Zarei and I. Saadat Akhtar
School of Veterinary Medicine, Shiraz University, Department of Clinical Studies, 7144169155, Iran; badiei33@gmail.com

Increasing the metabolic rate is an important effect of thyroid hormones and hence, these hormones are essential for body growth. The present study was conducted to clarify the normal levels of thyroid hormones and the effect of intravenous glucose on their circulating values in different periods (before and after parturition) in Iranian fat-tailed sheep. Five adult Iranian fat-tailed ewes were randomly selected and studied at 7 periods (4 and 2 weeks before parturition, 2 and 4 weeks and 2, 3 and 4 months after parturition). All sheep underwent the experiment, 2 h after the morning meal. At 0 h, dextrose 50% was intravenously administered at 500 mg/kg BW, 10 ml/kg/h. Jugular blood samples were taken at 0 h (before dextrose administration) and then 1, 2, 3 and 4 h thereafter and sera were immediately separated. Serum levels of glucose and thyroid hormones (T3 and T4) were assayed in all samples. Circulating levels of T3 were altered following intravenous glucose administration in all studied periods. The concentrations of T3 changed following administration of dextrose, at the different times realtive to lambing (2 weeks, 3 and 4 months after parturition) similarly increasing patterns of changes during the time after dextrose infusion were observed. At all stages, the lowest T3 concentration was seen at 0 h. The T3 concentrations changed following administration of dextrose at two and four weeks before parturition and had a similar decreasing pattern. For T4, no particular patterns of change were observed. Moreover, the circulating concentrations of the thyroid hormones were different in Iranian fat-tailed sheep during different physiological periods. Based on the effects of dextrose on these hormones, it may be suggested that glucose can affect the circulating thyroid hormone concentrations in sheep.

Comparing the economic impact of production diseases in dairy cattle between countries

M. Van Der Voort[1] and H. Hogeveen[1,2]
[1]Wageningen University, Business Economics Group, Hollandseweg 1, 6706 KN Wageningen, the Netherlands, [2]Utrecht University, 2Department of Farm Animal Health, Faculty of Veterinary Medicine, Yalelaan 7, 3584 CL Utrecht, the Netherlands; mariska.vandervoort@wur.nl

Production diseases cause large economic losses in dairy farming. Mastitis is reported as the most costly production disease in dairy cattle followed by fertility problems, lameness and metabolic disorders. A wide range of approaches and economic assessments have been published to calculate the economic impact of these production diseases. Examples of approaches vary from straightforward cost calculations to more complex bio-economic simulation models. These studies show large variations, which can be explained by the use of different data sources, assumptions that are taken, country specific variations and different calculation techniques. This makes it hardly impossible to compare the results of the different studies and to understand if differences in disease costs are due to the calculation methods or due to farms and country differences. The objective of this study is to compare the costs of production diseases between different dairy production systems and different countries. A calculation tool is developed considering general economic and technical farm data, like herds size, milk production and milk and feed prices. For each production disease (mastitis, lameness, metabolic disorders and reproduction problems), specific data on incidence, treatments, production effects and culling are collected. The disease costs were estimated by determining the milk production losses, discarded milk, treatments, veterinarian, farmers´ labor and death and culling. The data is based on literature and expert opinions, collected from the Netherlands, Florida (US), Minnesota (US) and New Zeeland. For each country a typical farm is defined. The total costs for the diseases varies substantially between countries and are highest for Florida, followed by Minnesota, New Zeeland and the Netherlands. However, the size of the average dairy herd in Florida is larger and therefore the disease costs per dairy cow are not always highest. The highest total costs are found for lameness, followed by reproduction disorders, mastitis and metabolic disorders. The biggest cost factors are losses in milk production and due to culling and death. For mastitis and reproduction disorders the size of the different costs factors varies a lot between the countries. In contrast to literature, we found that mastitis was not the most costly disease. The results stress out that the use of a standardized calculation method makes it possible to better understand the cost of disease between countries and production systems and allows to compare the different production diseases in a more structured way.

Economic impact of gastrointestinal parasitic infection on fattening of Desert Sheep

N. Eisa[1], S. Babiker[2] and H. Abdalla[3]
[1]University of Gezira, Department of Animal Production, Wad Medani, Gezira State, Sudan, [2]University of Khartoum, Department of Meat Production, Faculty of Animal Production, Khartoum North, Sudan, [3]University of Khartoum, Department of Parasitology, Faculty of Veterinary Medicine, Khartoum North, Sudan; eisanazk@yahoo.com

This study was conducted to evaluate the economic impact of natural gastrointestinal parasitic infection on fattening performance of Sudan Desert sheep. Forty-eight naturally infected lambs were divided into 2 groups of 24 lambs each. One group was treated for internal parasites while the other was left nturally infected. Each group was then divided into two groups according to age (old two years and young milk teeth) and dietary energy level (high and low). The design ended up with eight groups of 6 individuals each which were old treated high energy (OTHE), old infected high energy (OIHE), old treated low energy (OTLE), old infected low energy (OILE), young treated high energy (YTHE), young infected high energy (YIHE), young treated low energy (YTLE) and young infected low energy (YILE). They were then fattened for 60 days during which feedlot performance, mortality rate, purchase prices, sales and margins were calculated. The growth parameters as average daily gain and final body showed significantly ($P<0.001$) high differences among the treatments. Margin percent of sales of (OTHE) was 23.80% while (OILE) lost 40% of their total cost. Although (YTHE) ranked second in term of performance, but they achieved the best profit which was 5.7% more than the profit of (OTHE) because of less dry matter consumption. The number of sold lambs for (OILE) and (YILE) decreased by 50% due to mortality. Total margin of (OTHE) was 98.08 $, while (OIHE) was sold for 36.36% less profit. The earlier group gained 82.81% more profit than (OTLE). Although older treated lambs gained more weight than younger ones but economically younger lambs were more profitable. Total sales revenue of (OTHE) was 510 $ with 19.2% total margin, while the total sales revenue of (YTHE) was 480 $ reaching 24.9% total margin. Concentrate supplementation policy has to be followed to increase productivity of sheep and to lower mortality due to gastrointestinal parasites specially when in poor rainy seasons. Governments has to adopt such policy to protect the national grazing herd. More studies about the effect of gastrointestinal parasites on sheep need to be conducted.

Impact of different production systems on health care costs in the Dutch broiler farms

E. Gocsik, H.E. Kortes, A.G.J.M. Oude Lansink and H.W. Saatkamp
Wageningen University, Business Economics Group, Hollandseweg 1, 6706 KN Wageningen, the Netherlands; eva.gocsik@wur.nl

In recent years, increasing requirements regarding animal welfare in broiler production have led to the development of production systems that comply with above-legal animal welfare standards. The aim of this study was to analyze the impact of different production systems, including the conventional and five alternative production systems, on health care costs. Firstly, we investigated whether higher animal welfare standards increased health care costs in both absolute and relative terms. Secondly, we examined which cost components (losses or expenditures) were affected and to what extent. This study was restricted to the most important endemic diseases, i.e. infectious bronchitis, coccidiosis, *E. coli*, necrotic enteritis, infectious bursal disease, sudden death syndrome, ascites, and leg problems. Production and health care costs were calculated for each delivered broiler in an Excel model using the partial budgeting approach. Three categories of production systems were distinguished based on the results concerning health care costs. The first category includes conventional systems, in which diseases affecting the gastrointestinal tract and leg problems had the highest impact on production costs in both absolute and relative terms. Production costs per delivered broiler increased by €0.144 in case of *E. coli* and by €0.071 in case of necrotic enteritis. Similarly, in the second category (incl. Volwaard, Better Life 1*, and Better Life 2* systems), gastrointestinal diseases and leg problems had the highest impact on production costs. However, the impact of these diseases was lower than that of diseases in conventional system. The decrease in impact can be explained by the fact that these AW systems use a more robust breed with a slower growth rate. In the third category (incl. Better Life 3*, and organic systems), gastrointestinal diseases had the highest impact and the overall impact of gastrointestinal diseases was similar to that in the conventional system. However, the impact of coccidiosis increased compared to the conventional system, most likely due to prohibition on the use of anticoccidial drugs and the provision of an outdoor access. Moreover, leg problems and heart and vascular diseases disappeared completely. We conclude that, losses account for the major part of health care costs, which makes it difficult to detect the actual impact of diseases on total health care costs. Besides, although differences in health care costs exist across production systems, health care costs only make a minor contribution to the total production costs relative to other costs, such as feed costs and purchase of day-old chicks.

Economic losses due to subclinical ketosis and related disorders in dairy herds of Iran

M. Sakha[1] and S. Nejat Dehkordi[2]
[1]Science and Research Branch, Islamic Azad University, Clinical Sciences, Faculty of Specialized Veterinary Sciences, Ashrafi highway, Hesarak, 14515-755 Tehran, Iran, [2]Sharkord branch, Islamic Azad University, School of Veterinary Medicine, Sharkord, 14321, Iran; msakha@yahoo.com

Ketosis is a major production disease of modern agriculture that causes of loss to the dairy herds and the main economic loss is due to the loss of production while the disease is present and failure to return to full production after recovery. The transition from late gestation, non-lactating to non pregnant, lactating presents significant challenges to the cow's system. When nutrition management does not meet these challenges, a wide range of health problems can result. Metabolic diseases are disorders that originally are nutritional and often result in acute symptoms requiring treatment. A total of two hundred-three multiparous Holstein cows (parity 2-9) were randomly selected of ten industrial dairy farms. Blood samples were investigated for BHB concentration in one week before, two weeks and three weeks after parturition. The relation of subclinical ketosis(SCK) and peripartum disorders also were considered and economic losses were calculated. Using cut-off 1,200 umol/l for BHB concentration the frequency of subclinical ketosis was 13.79%. There was a significant correlation between SCK and LDA(odds ratio 9.74) metritis (odds ratio 4.260 and mastitis (odds ratio 6.64). Economic loss for SCK alone was nearly 41.4 $ per head and considering related disorders it will reach about 320, 150 and 190 $ per head for LDA, metritis and mastitis respectively. Regarding the considerable prevalence of SCK in dairy herd under study there is high economic losses in dairy herd in Iran. The prevalence of SCK in other parts of Iran are reported equally. So preventive methods in relation to periparturient disorders is important. While there are some traces for abnormal biochemicals in some of animals, hence, push for more production in animals that are not much suited for this purpose is an important question production of some disorders related to alterations in diet due to complex situations such as drop in intake or some social/environmental effects are not enough documents for more manipulation of style of life of the animal. In conclusion, more investigation should be done to evaluate the animal potentials for alteration of living status that goes for animal welfare.

Economic decision-making on reducing risks of human exposure to AMR through livestock supply chains

J.L. Roskam[1], E. Gocsik[1], A.G.J.M. Oude Lansink[1], M.L.W. Schut[2,3] and H.W. Saatkamp[1]
[1]Wageningen University, Social Sciences, Business Economics Group, P.O. Box 8130, 6700 EW Wageningen, the Netherlands, [2]International Institute of Tropical Agriculture (IITA), Quartier Kabondo, Rohero 1, Avenue 18 Septembre 10, Bujumbura, Burundi, [3]Wageningen University, Social Sciences, Knowledge, Technology and Innovation Group, P.O. Box 8130, 6700 EW Wageningen, the Netherlands; jamal.roskam@wur.nl

Antimicrobial resistance is one of the biggest threats for both human and animal health. The aim of this research was to provide a comprehensive supply chain based conceptual framework that includes an inventory of all main measures and strategies that could affect the risks of human exposure to antimicrobial resistance. Such an inventory is essential in the process of decision-making surrounding the problem of antimicrobial resistance, particularly from an economic decision-making point of view. The focus in this conceptualization is on the prevalence of resistant (pathogenic) microorganisms in food animals and products, originating from broiler and pig supply chains, through which humans can be exposed to antimicrobial resistance. The conceptual framework consists of two parts. The first part elaborates on the main measures and strategies, both on-farm and beyond-farm, and includes both antimicrobial and non-antimicrobial related measures and strategies. The second part of the framework covers the aspect of (non-)compliance behaviour and effectivity of measures and strategies. Most on-farm measures and strategies can influence the microbial population in food animals by affecting the prevalence of (pathogenic) microorganisms and the ratio between antimicrobial resistant and non-resistant (pathogenic) microorganisms. That ratio remains unaffected after the slaughtering process, but the absolute prevalence and counting's can still be influenced, either negatively through factors that can cause an increase in prevalence, like cross-contamination, or positively through measures and strategies that can decrease the prevalence of (pathogenic) microorganisms, like different decontamination treatments. It is concluded that the conceptualization provides a sound basis for economic decision-support to policymakers. In addition, the conceptual framework should constitute the qualitative basis for future bio-economic model development and other quantitative analyses that can result in policy guidelines that support the process of economic decision-making surrounding the problem of antimicrobial resistance.

The devastating effects of foot-and-mouth disease in dairy farm

A. Hayirli[1], M. Cengiz[2], M.O. Timurkan[3], S. Cengiz[4], B. Balli[1] and F. Hira[1]
[1]Atatürk University, Faculty of Veterinary Medicine, Department of Animal Nutrition & Nutritional Disorders, 25240 Erzurum, Turkey, [2]Atatürk University, Faculty of Veterinary Medicine, Department of Obstetrics and Gynecology, 25240 Erzurum, Turkey, [3]Atatürk University, Faculty of Veterinary Medicine, Department of Virology, 25240 Erzurum, Turkey, [4]Atatürk University, Faculty of Veterinary Medicine, Department of Microbiology, 25240 Erzurum, Turkey; ahayirli_2000@yahoo.com

The aim of this study was to summarize 2-lactation performance of pregnant Fleckvieh heifers imported from Austria to a dairy farm located in Northeastern Turkey in 2013. The mean days in pregnancy at the time of arrival was 190.4±30.2 (129-245, n=119). Despite vaccinating with a trivalent vaccine (A, O, Asia1) 15 days after arrival, all animals were affected by foot-and-mouth disease (FMD, O type) 2.5 months after arrival. The mortality rate as well as production and reproduction data were subjected to descriptive statistics. The mortality rate was 29.4, 4.8, and 10% at around 1st parturition (35/119) and in the 1st lactation (4/84) and 2nd lactation (8/80) cycles, respectively. Deaths at around 1st partition were related to FMD and its complications (lameness, n=48; mastitis, n=42) (8 at 268.0±9.8 days in pregnancy and 27 at 21.2±28.1 days in milk), whereas 4 and 8 cows were culled due to infertility and traumatic injury at the 1st and 2nd lactation cycles. 111, 81 and 74 cows delivered 112, 85, and 78 calves, and of these, 67 (59%), 5 (5.8%), and 6 (7.6%) calves died at the 1st, 2nd, and 3rd parturition, respectively. Calves at 1st parturition died within 3 days due to abortion and cardiomyopathy resulting from FMD. The mean days in milk, days in dry, days open, artificial insemination per pregnancy, daily milk yield, 305-d milk production, and calving interval were 367±74 (242-565), 79±45 (40-264), 164±86 (38-459), 3.09±1.69 (1-9), 13.4±3.3 (7.2-20.6), 4,089±997 (2186-6272), and 447±86 (307-748) at the 1st lactation cycle (n=80) and 300±62 (113-471), 74±49 (8-338), 89±57 (35-262), 2.03±1.21 (1-7), 19.7±4.9 (9.0-30.0), 6,015±1493 (2745-9150), and 373±61 (280-562) at the 2nd lactation cycle (n=72), respectively. The data suggest that in addition to completion of infrastructure, importers should receive education and technical support on animal husbandry before arrival of animals, especially FMD-free countries to contaminated countries.

Economic weights for health traits in livestock

M. Michaličková, Z. Krupová, E. Krupa and L. Zavadilová
Institute of Animal Science, Přátelství 815, 104 00 Prague 10, Czech Republic;
michalickova.monika@vuzv.cz

Health traits have an impact on the profitability through effective utilisation of inputs, reduction of costs, improvement of milk price, and security of production. Therefore, more attention has been recently paid to their genetic improvement. Economic values for the complex of health traits (somatic cells score, productive lifetime of cows, claw disease incidence and clinical mastitis incidence, ect.) in dairy production system of Slovak Simmental (SS) and Slovak Pinzgau (SP) cattle were calculated. The bio-economic model of the program package ECOWEIGHT 6.0.4 (for cattle) was used for calculation. At present, the module for pigs (EWPIG) is under development. Similarly as in cattle, health traits are included when calculating economic values of traits. Under the production and economic conditions of the period 2011-2013, somatic cells score (12.5% on average) and productive lifetime of cows (10.9% on average) were found as the most important traits in both cattle breeds. The marginal economic value of somatic cell score was -497.2 and -241.1 €/score per cow and year in SS and SP breed, respectively. The appropriate economic values for production lifetime were 105.54 and 76.4 €/year per cow and year, respectively. Considering the direct health traits, the incidence of clinical mastitis were of higher economic importance (-63.9 and -70.7 € per case per cow per year) compared to the claw diseases incidence (-22.8 and -26.7 € per case per cow per year for SS and SP breed, respectively). Moreover for the last mentioned traits, the lowest relative importance (1.1% and 0.2%, respectively) among all of the evaluated traits was calculated. The differences between marginal and relative importance of health traits were associated with the average milk production (e. g. somatic cells count content in kg of milk) and economic parameters (e. g. level of costs and revenues) of evaluated breeds. Generally, increase in mean value of health traits is economically unfavourable (e. g. due to discarding of milk during cow illness as well as due to additional costs for drugs, veterinary service and labour for herdsman and veterinary time). Based on the current status, results found in this study provide the first information important for further development of the selection indices of the local breeds with regards to health traits. Furthermore, the growing interest of consumers in socio-ethical aspects of animal production thought the non-economic value of health traits should be taken into account. This study was funded by the project QJ1510217, QJ1310109 and MZERO0714 of the Czech Republic.

Occurrences of production diseases in grower pigs on Irish pig farms

N. Van Staaveren[1,2], B. Doyle[2], A. Hanlon[1] and L. Boyle[2]
[1]University College Dublin, School of Veterinary Medicine, Belfield, Dublin 4, Ireland, [2]Teagasc Animal and Grassland Research and Innovation Centre, Pig Development Department, Moorepark, Fermoy, Co. Cork, Ireland; bernadette.doyle@teagasc.ie

Nutritional and management factors play an important role in maintaining pigs' health and welfare. This study aimed to identify production diseases in each of the different production stages of Irish grower pigs. Preliminary findings on the prevalence of identified production diseases are presented. An adapted Welfare Quality® protocol was conducted on 31 integrated pigs farms (July-November 2015). Eighteen pens were randomly selected across 1st stage weaner, 2nd stage weaner and finisher pigs per farm (n=6 per stage). Pens were observed for 10 min and number of pigs with the following conditions was recorded: poor body condition (PBC), dead, sick (i.e. listless/laboured breathing), twisted snout, rectal prolapse, hernia, skin and neurological conditions, eye infections and lameness. These conditions were expressed as average percentage of pigs in a pen affected (mean ± SE) and were ranked to identify the three most common conditions for each production stage. In 1st stage pens the most commonly observed condition was PBC with 5.2±0.4% of pigs affected (range: 0-30%), followed by pigs showing signs of sickness (1.7±0.2%; range: 0-18.2%) and hernias (umbilical: 0.4±0.1%; range: 0-18.2%; scrotal: 0.6±0.1%; range: 0-7.1%). PBC was also the most commonly observed condition in 2nd stage pens (2.0±0.2%; range: 0-12.5%) but with a lower proportion of pigs affected compared to the 1st stage. Hernias were the second most common condition (umbilical: 1.0±0.2%; range: 0-15.3%; scrotal: 0.7±0.1%; range: 0-16.7%) followed by lameness (1.0±0.2%; range: 0-16.7%). In the finisher stage, hernias were the most commonly observed condition (umbilical: 1.8±0.2%; range: 0-12.5%; scrotal: 0.4±0.1%; range: 0-10.5%). Lameness was the second most commonly observed condition (1.3±0.2%; range: 0-15.4%) and PBC the third (1.1±0.2%; range: 0-12.5%). Consistent with nutritional challenges associated with weaning, PBC was the most commonly observed condition in weaner pens. Weaning stress could also explain why sick pigs were only seen in the top three conditions for pigs in the 1st stage pens. As the pigs got older hernias and lameness became more common reflecting problems potentially associated with high growth rates and heavier body weights. Large variation existed between pens for all conditions with the prevalence of health conditions in certain pens/farms posing concerns for pig welfare. These preliminary results show that occurrences of production diseases recorded reflected the different challenges pigs face at each production stage.

Associations between tail lesions and lung health in slaughter pigs

N. Van Staaveren[1,2], A. Vale[1], E.G. Manzanilla[2], B. Doyle[2], A. Hanlon[1] and L. Boyle[2]
[1]University College Dublin, School of Veterinary Medicine, Belfield, Dublin 4, Ireland, [2]Teagasc Animal and Grassland Research and Innovation Centre, Pig Development Department, Moorepark, Fermoy, Co. Cork, Ireland; nienke.vanstaaveren@teagasc.ie

Tail lesions are important indicators of pig welfare and are potential 'iceberg indicators' capable of providing information on the overall health and welfare of pigs. Tail lesions can be associated with poor health directly by providing a route of entry for pathogens or indirectly through shared risk factors for tail biting and disease. This study investigated associations between carcass tail lesion and lung lesion severity scores in slaughter pigs in order to evaluate the use of carcass tail lesions as indicators of lung health. Abattoir visits occurred over 5 days (January-March 2015). Tail lesion score (0-4) according to severity, sex, and kill number was recorded for every pig after scalding and dehairing. Lungs from each carcass were scored for lesions using an adapted version of the BPEX pig health scheme. Severity of pleurisy was scored on a 0 to 2 scale with score 2 equating to severe pleurisy or lungs attached to the chest wall ('lungs in chest'). The database for assessing pleurisy lesions contained all pleurisy scores (n=5,628). However, lungs with a score 2 for pleurisy could not be assessed for other lesions and were excluded from analysis of all other lung lesions (n=4,491). Associations between tail lesions and sex and the different lung lesion outcomes were analysed using generalized linear mixed models (PROC GLIMMIX) with random effect for batch. Prevalence of EP-like lesions (58.1%; range 23.1-90.1%) and pleurisy (42.6%; range 4.4-80.2%) was high though large variation was observed between batches. No association was found between tail lesion severity and occurrence of diseased lungs, EP categories, or pleurisy categories (*P*>0.05). However, tail lesion score tended to be associated with retention of lungs in the carcass due to severe pleurisy ('lungs in chest'; *P*=0.1). This retention of lungs was observed more often in pigs with severe tail lesions than in pigs with moderate tail lesions (OR=4.1; 95% CI 1.10-15.15; *P*=0.09). Tail lesions on the carcass may not be an accurate predictor of lung health in individual pigs. However, due to shared risk factors, batch level analysis may reveal significant associations between tail lesion and lung disease prevalence. Further research is also needed to elucidate the relationship between severe pleurisy (lungs in chest) and tail lesion susceptibility. Both tail lesions and respiratory disease have significant economic and welfare implications and recording these conditions during meat inspection can provide information regarding on-farm health/welfare of pigs.

Relationship between 'pig flow' from birth to slaughter and the risk of disease at slaughter

J. Calderon-Diaz[1], L.A. Boyle[1], A. Diana[1,2], F.C. Leonard[2], M. Mcelroy[3], S. Mcgettrick[3], J. Moriarty[3] and E.G. Manzanilla[1]

[1]Teagasc, Pig Development Department, Animal and Grassland Research and Innovation Centre, Moorepark, Fermoy, Co. Cork, Ireland, [2]School of Veterinary Medicine, University College Dublin, Belfield, Dublin 4, Ireland, [3]Central Veterinary Research Laboratory, Backweston Campus, Celbridge, Co. Kildare, Ireland; julia.calderondiaz@teagasc.ie

The flow of pigs through a unit on an 'all in-all out' basis is crucial in the control of disease. The aim of this study was to determine the relationship between different frequencies of detention of pigs during the production cycle on carcass weight and the risk of pericarditis, heart condemnations and lameness at slaughter. A batch of pigs (n=1045) born during one week in a commercial integrated herd were followed after tagging and weighing at birth through to slaughter. On the day prior to slaughter the pigs locomotory ability was scored on a three point scale as 0 (normal) or ≥1 (lame). The presence or absence of pericarditis was recorded at the point of viscera inspection where heart condemnations were also recorded on the basis of the decision of the acting veterinary inspector. In a nested case control study matching by weight (pigs between 4 and 7 kg) 76 pigs retained once (O) and 52 pigs retained several (S) times were compared to 185 pigs following an uninterrupted (U) pig flow. The relationship of sow parity, no. of movements during lactation, no. of times animals were retained with carcass weights (mixed models) and the occurrence of pericarditis, heart condemnation and lameness (logistic regression) was studied. S pigs had lower carcass weights (76.9±1.41 kg) than U (85.5±0.87 kg) or O (87.8±1.19 kg pigs ($P<0.05$). S pigs also had higher odds of having a heart condemned (OR 3.54, CI: 1.44, 8.73; $P<0.01$) and of pericarditis (OR 3.13, CI: 1.28, 7.65; $P<0.05$) relative to U pigs. Both S (OR 5.51, CI 2.41, 12.57) and O (OR 3.74, CI 1.71, 8.19) pigs had higher odds of being lame ($P<0.001$). Pigs born to sows of parities 3 and 4 had lower odds of being lame ($P<0.05$) while pigs born to sows of parities 5 and 6 tended to have lower odds of being lame ($P<0.10$). The higher likelihood of heart disease in pigs that did not follow an 'all-in all out' pattern of pig flow supports the theory that this practice is associated with the re-circulation of disease. Further analysis will elucidate whether the findings regarding lameness and carcass weight are causative or explanatory. These findings also suggest that pigs born to gilts might be at greater risk of lameness.

A novel scoring system for the classification of the health status of growing-finishing pig farms

A.J.M. Jansman[1], E. Kampman-Van De Hoek[1,2], P. Sakkas[2], H. Van Beers-Schreurs[3], C.M.C. Van Der Peet-Schwering[1], J.J.G.C. Van Den Borne[2] and W.J.J. Gerrits[2]

[1]Wageningen UR Livestock Research, Animal Nutrition, P.O. Box 338, 6700 AH Wageningen, the Netherlands, [2]Wageningen University, Animal Nutrition Group, P.O. Box 338, 6700 AH Wageningen, the Netherlands, [3]Veterinary Medicines Authority (SDa), Yalelaan 114, 3584 CM Utrecht, the Netherlands; alfons.jansman@wur.nl

Health status of pig farms can vary considerably and relates to the variation in zootechnical performance among farms. Classification of farm health can be helpful in monitoring farm health status in time and for the application of intervention strategies to improve farm health status. The aim of the current study was to develop a concept for classification of the health status of growing-finishing pig farms. Six traits were incorporated into a health status web, related to the zootechnical performance and measurements at slaughter. Performance data from 1,074 and 783 Dutch pig farms, and abattoir data of 50,208 and 47,426 farm deliveries to slaughterhouses, acquired over 2011 and 2012 respectively, were used as a representative sample for the Dutch growing-finishing pig population to calculate the 25th and 75th percentiles of each trait per year. Per farm, a score was calculated per trait by inter- and extrapolation using the 25th and 75th percentiles from the Dutch pig population. The farm score was defined as the mean score over the six traits. A farm was classified as having a suboptimal health with a farm score between 50 and 62.5, as having a conventional health status with a farm score between 62.5 and 87.5 and as having a high health status with a farm score between 87.5 and 100. Further, two datasets were compiled: dataset 1 with farm data of 179 farms over the year 2011, and dataset 2 with farm data of 70 farms over both 2011 and 2012. In dataset 1, 13 farms were characterized as high health, 159 farms as conventional and seven farms as having a low health status. Analysis of dataset 2 revealed that farm scores are consistent across years, indicating that the farm score is farm specific and the health status web is a valuable concept to characterize growing-finishing pig farms on their health status.

Management factors associated with mortality of dairy calves

L. Seppä-Lassila[1], K. Sarjokari[1,2], M. Hovinen[1], T. Soveri[1] and M. Norring[1]
[1]University of Helsinki, Department of Production Animal Medicine, P.O. Box 57, 00014 University of Helsinki, Finland, [2]Valio Ltd, P.O. Box 10, 00039 Valio, Finland; leena.seppa-lassila@helsinki.fi

Mortality of dairy calves can reflect suboptimal production environment or management, and can be considered as a crude indicator of overall calf welfare. We aimed to identify potential management factors that affect calf mortality in order to eventually help reducing calf mortality. Mortality data of 13,580 calves from 82 farms with average herd size of 125±41 cows were acquired from Finnish Agricultural data processing center. Data on management practices were collected during farm visits by interviewing farmers with a structured questionnaire. The calf mortality data were analyzed using linear regression models. At the herd level, the mean mortality of calves that were less than 7 days of age, was 5.2±2.3%. Every increase of 10 cows in herd size increased mortality rate by 0.13 percentage points ($P=0.019$). Separating sick calves from healthy ones decreased the mortality rate by 1.38 percentage point ($P=0.005$). In addition, higher mortality tended to be associated with longer latency from birth until colostrum intake (0.13 percentage point increase for every one hour delay; $P=0.083$), lower average parity (1.72 percentage point increase in mortality rate for every one parity decrease in the mean; $P=0.097$) and a smaller proportion of breeds other than Ayrshire or Holstein in the herd (0.29 percentage point decrease for every percentage point decrease in breed proportions; $P=0.053$). The mean mortality of older calves aged 7 to 180 days was 5.7±6.2%. Mortality rate increased with a shorter whole milk feeding period (0.01 percentage point increase for every one day shorter period; $P=0.008$), longer period in the calving pen (0.19 percentage point increase for every one day; $P=0.016$), and smaller average herd production level (0.32 percentage point increase by every 1000 kg decrease in average milk yield; $P=0.001$). Mortality of calves was 0.39 percentage point lower on farms that used a veterinarian to disbud calves instead of farmer/other person ($P=0.024$). In addition, mortality tended to be lower on farms which sold lower proportion of calves (0.008 percentage point decrease by every percentage point increase of proportion of calves sold; $P=0.065$) and that had natural ventilation instead of forced (0.47 percentage point decrease, $P=0.071$). More attentive management procedures; advancing health by colostrum feeding, separating sick calves, and using a veterinarian for disbudding can help reducing calf mortality rate on farm. Larger farms, farms with smaller average production and farms with lower average parity had higher calf mortality rates. Particular consideration should be used on these farms when tackling mortality issues.

Network for evaluation of One Health: working together for improved health of the global community

J. Starič[1], F. Farci[2] and B. Häsler[3]
[1]University of Ljubljana, Veterinary faculty, Gerbičeva 60, 1000 Ljubljana, Slovenia, [2]University of Sassari, Piazza Università 21, Sassari, Italy, [3]Royal Veterinary College, Hawkshead Lane, North Mymms, Hatfield AL9 7TA, United Kingdom; joze.staric@vf.uni-lj.si

The problems linked to global changes associated with human health, malnutrition, animal health, climate, emergence of new zoonosis and endemic/epidemic diseases cannot be understood and tackled using disciplinary methods only. The complexity of these issues requires a global transdisciplinary and multi-sectoral approach to understand the dynamics and underlying mechanisms of the events that characterize them, and to obtain optimal solutions for economically sustainable risk management. Founded by a new Trans Domain Action of the European Program 'COST' the 'Network for Evaluation of One Health' (NEOH) (http://neoh.onehealthglobal.net) (TD1404) provides the opportunity for European countries (currently 22 COST countries and 4 international partner countries), professionals and scientists who work in different disciplines (e.g. ecology, economics, human and animal health, epidemiology, social sciences, etc.) not only to network and exchange information, but also to learn about different global health critical points of relevance to the sectors and to discuss systemic approaches to health and their evaluation. This allows us to generate a holistic vision and to contribute to solutions that improve health of the global community. Participants in NEOH work together in four different Working Groups (WGs). The purpose of the first (WG1) is to enable quantitative evaluations of One Health (OH) by developing a standardized evaluation protocol to be applied in a suite of case studies. The next step is to apply in WG2 the protocol in OH cases/projects to test the approach proposed. WG3 will conduct a meta-analysis of the available case study results to facilitate international comparison and the elaboration of policy recommendations. Finally, WG4 targets to establish contacts through meetings and conferences within the NEOH consortium, but also with external relevant stakeholders to get their input and feedback. This network runs from 2014 to 2018 and is open to anybody engaged in One Health and its evaluation.

Epidemiological study of growth performance and carcass quality in pigs fed a low or high complexity

H. Reinhardt, C.F.M. De Lange and V. Farzan
University of Guelph, Department of Animal Biosciences and Department of Population Medicine, 50 Stone Road, N1G 2W1, Canada; hreinhar@uoguelph.ca

Feed is the main cost of pork production. Feeding pigs less complex and less expensive nursery diets will compromise growth performance during the nursery phase, but may induce compensatory growth thereafter and reduce production costs. The objective of this study was to investigate effects of using a low complexity (LC; containing reduced animal protein) nursery pig feeding program on subsequent growth performance and carcass quality. On each of seven commercial farms, 60 piglets were selected from 8 to 10 sows within 24 to 96 h after birth and identified by an ear tag. Pigs were weighed five times: at birth, at weaning, and at the end of nursery, grower and finisher phases. The study was conducted twice on each farm. At weaning, the pigs were assigned to two dietary treatments: LC vs high complexity (HC) nursery feeding program. Carcass quality information (back fat depth, loin eye depth and lean yield) was collected for all pigs at slaughter. A survey was conducted to determine pig density, pig flow, in-feed medication, vaccination, diseases history and mortality, as well as sow productivity including parity, litter size at birth, and live born. A multilevel mixed-effect linear regression modeling method was used to analyze average daily gain, body weight, and carcass quality. The mean average daily gains (kg) (HC vs LC, respectively) was 0.244 vs 0.239 (suckling), 0.428 vs 0.417 (nursery), 0.828 vs 0.836 (grower), and 1.036 vs 1.042 (finisher); while mean body weight (kg) were 1.9 vs 1.9 (after birth), 7.1 vs 6.9 (at weaning), 24.3 vs 23.8 (at end of nursery), 60.6 vs 60.2 (at end of grower), and 105.1 vs 104.7 (at end of finisher). Mean back fat depth (mm), loin eye depth (mm), and lean yield (%) were 20.4, 68.4 and 60.3 for HC and 20.8, 67.6 and 60.2 for LC, respectively. Multivariable analysis with farm as random effect suggested that average daily gain of pigs on LC was not different from that of pigs on HC ($P>0.05$). However, mean age at slaughter for HC (175.5 days) was higher than that for LC (173.8 days ($P=0.04$). Mixed-level regression analysis with farm and pig as random effect showed that there was no effect of dietary treatment on body weight of pigs at all phases and on carcass characteristics ($P>0.05$). Nursery pigs can be fed a reduced complexity feeding program without negative impacts on growth performance up to slaughter weight and carcass quality. Further research is required to ensure the pigs susceptibility to disease is not compromised by feeding LC nursery diets.

Induced copper deficiency in a sheep flock

R.J. Van Saun
Pennsylvania State University, Veterinary & Biomedical Sciences, 115 Henning Building, 16802, USA; rjv10@psu.edu

This presentation is a case study where copper deficiency presented as stillborn and weak, dying lambs with 2-year old ewe losses. The objective is to describe a diagnostic approach in defining the underlying issue and an approach to correct the problem. The case study farms raise sheep for meat production and are managed by a father (Farm A) and daughter (Farm B) on two adjacent, but separate properties in western Pennsylvania. The two flocks consist of 100 and 60 ewes of Texel and Suffolk breeds with over 180% lambing percentage. Animals are extensively managed and fed on pasture for more than 7 months of the year. When pasture is not available, harvested hay from each respective farm is fed in addition to 450 g/d of a custom energy and protein supplement for late pregnant ewes. A trace mineral salt product is available free choice on pasture and in lambing barns. Lambing occurred on both farms between February and March. No issues were present on Farm A during the 2015 lambing season, while Farm B experienced severe lamb and ewe losses with 2-year old ewes. Older ewes were unaffected and had live lambs. Farm B lost 24 of 25 2-year old ewes with no lamb survivals. All lambs from these ewes were either stillborn or died soon after birth. Affected ewes first presented as lethargic and within 24-48 h were found dead. Diagnostic samples of lamb and ewe mortalities were submitted to the Animal Diagnostic Laboratory at Pennsylvania State University for a flock workup. Feed ingredient analyses were collected, sent for analysis and results are presented on a dry matter (DM) basis. Stillborn lambs and ewes submitted to the diagnostic laboratory showed no gross abnormalities on necropsy and no positive microbiologic findings. Stillborn lambs had liver Cu concentrations between 14.7 and 22.2 µg/g (reference: 25-100 µg/g wet weight). Hepatic zinc (11.5 and 48.5 µg/g; reference: 30-75 µg/g) and vitamin E (1.0 and 1.7 µg/g; reference: 5-50 µg/g) were also low or marginal in these lambs. Dead ewes had normal hepatic Cu (140 µg/g; reference: 88-400 µg/g dry weight), but highly elevated Mo (6.68 µg/g; reference: 1.4-3.2 µg/g dry weight). Affected surviving sheep were either moved and fed at Farm A or administered a 2 gm CuO bolus. Subsequent serum Cu concentrations showed differences, but improved Cu status. This was an unusual clinical presentation of Cu deficiency with aborted or stillborn lambs and ewe deaths, which are not commonly considered a consequence of Cu deficiency. High concentration of forage Mo (>6 ppm DM) relative to Cu (<13 ppm DM) was responsible for low dietary Cu availability. Forages should be evaluated for Mo and S status in evaluating level of dietary Cu supplementation to ensure adequate availability.

Effect of restricted feeding on rumen fermentation of Japanese Black fattening steers during summer

Y. Maeda[1,2], K. Nishimura[2] and S. Kushibiki[1,3]
[1]*Tsukuba University, Graduate School of Life and Environmental Sciences, Tsukuba, 305-8577, Japan,* [2]*Miyazaki Livestock Research Institute, Takaharu, 889-4411, Japan,* [3]*Nationl Institute of Livestock and Grassland Science, Tsukuba, 305-0901, Japan; maeda-yuka@pref.miyazaki.lg.jp*

Japanese Black fattening cattle are generally fed concentrates ad libitum that contain large amounts of volatile carbohydrates, such as starch. However, ingestion of large amounts of starch disturbs homeostasis in the rumen environment, resulting in a high risk of metabolism disorders. Furthermore, several studies have shown that heat stress during summer affects body weight gain and dry matter intake of livestock. Feeding concentrates ad libitum during summer could lead to deterioration in feed efficiency caused by rumen fermentation. In the present study, the effect of restricted feeding on digestibility and rumen fermentation of Japanese Black fattening steers during summer was examined. Eight 26-month-old Japanese Black steers were divided into two groups. The restricted group (RG, n=4) was fed concentrate and rice straw with the ratio of total digestible nutrients (TDN) 110% to of the Japanese Feeding Standard for fattening steer, expecting a daily gain of 0.75 kg. The control group (CG, n=4) was supplied both concentrate and rice straw ad libitum. In the experiment 1 (Exp. 1), dry matter intake (DMI) and nutrient intake were measured via the total faces collection method, and volatile fatty acid (VFA) concentration and rumen endotoxin were measured via the rumen juice orally collected. In the experiment 2 (Exp. 2), ruminal pH in both groups (n=3, respectively) was measured continuously every 10 minutes using a radio-transmission pH-measurement senser (Yamagata TOA DKK Co., Japan). Both experiments were carried out in July and/or August 2015. Temperature, relative humidity, and temperature-humidity index (THI) were 26.9°, 82.5%, and 78.2, respectively, during the experimental period. There was no significant difference in DMI between both groups; however, digestibility of dry matter (DM), organic matter (OM), crude protein (CP), and neutral detergent fiber (NDF) were significantly higher in RG than those in CG. VFA concentration was significantly lower in RG. However, there were no significant differences in VFA composition and endotoxin activity between both groups. Average ruminal pH was significantly lower in RG then in CG in the experimental period. Ruminal pH before morning feeeding (8:00) was significantly higher in CG for 21 h (9:00-5:00), and for 14 h (10:00-23:00) in RG. Total hours ruminal pH lower than the before morning feeding par day was lesser in RG than in CG. These results suggest that restricted feeding of Japanese Black fattening steers during summer could improve rumen function via increase forage digestibility.

Evaluation of serum passive transfer status in calves and colostrum with the Brix refractometer

H. Batmaz and O. Topal

Faculty of Veterinary Medicine, Veterinary Internal Medicine, Uludag University, Animal Hospital, Görükle Campus, Nilüfer/BURSA, 16059, Turkey; onurtopal@uludag.edu.tr

Passive transfer (PT) is very important for health of neonatal calves. For good PT, colostrum should be of good quality and it should be given to the calf as soon as possible with sufficient volume. The objective of this study was to evaluate relationships between percentage Brix digital refractometer (colostrum and calf serum) and serum total protein (TP), gamma glutamyltransferase (GGT) and glutaraldehyde coagulation time (GCT) in first three days. In this study, colostrum of 28 calving Holstein (2.5-7 years old) cows and serum of 29 calves born from these cows are used as materials. Calves had drunk first colostrum by bottle nipples within 3 h after birth. They drank approximately 2-2.5 lt colostrum twice daily on first three days. Percentage of Brix were measured of colostrum (first-milking, first day and second day). Percentage of Brix, TP, GGT and GCT in serum of calves were determined before drinking colostrum (day 0), and on the first day and third day. Significant differences were determined on three different days for all parameters ($P<0.05$). A positive correlation was found between percentage of Brix on calves before colostrum drinking and TP, and a negative correlation between percentage of Brix on calves and GGT. First-milking colostrum quality was found as 61.53% excellent, 26.92% good and 11.53% weak, according to the reference value of the Brix instrument. It was observed that calves were 48.27% excellent PT, 34.48% good PT, 17.24% of failure PT (FPT) on first day and 68.9% excellent PT, 13.79% good PT, 17.24% FPT on third day according to percentage Brix serum. Correlation was observed between percentage Brix serum and TP (highly), GGT and GCT (moderately) on first and third day. Except for five calves with FPT, a correlation was found between percentage Brix of first-milking colostrum and percentage of Brix serum and TP on first day. Although five calves suckled good-excellent Brix value of colostrum, FPT may develop inadequate intake (volume) of colostrum. As a result in the first three days, it was observed that the percentage brix of colostrum reflects the quality of colostrum, and a good correlation was found between percentage of brix serum and TP, GGT, GCT for assesment of PT in calves.

Effects of vitamin and element supplementation on weight gain of calves fed raw or pasteurised milk

Z. Mecitoglu and H. Batmaz

Uludag University, Faculty of Veterinary Medicine, Dep. of Internal Medicine, Görükle Kampüsü, 16059 Bursa, Turkey; zafer_mo@hotmail.com

Pasteurisation of milk, fed to calves is recommended for the control of some diseases in dairy herds. However pasteurisation of milk is demonstrated to decrease levels of Vitamin B1, B12, C and E. Also levels of trace elements such as Fe, Cu and Zn could be negatively influenced by heat treatment of raw milk as demonstrated by Zurera-Cosano *et al.* Aim of the presented study was to investigate the effects of commercial milk supplement (Milkshake®, Mervue Lab., Ireland) containing vitamins and trace elements, on weight gain and basic health status of dairy calves. The study was conducted on 40 calves from two different herds. Ten calves from herd A received raw milk and 7.5 g of the milk supplement twice daily for 60 days (Group AM); 10 other calves did not receive any treatment and were fed with raw milk for 60 days (Group AC). Calves from herd B were divided into two groups, Group BM (n:10) received 7.5 g of the milk supplement twice daily for 60 days mixed with flash pasteurised milk (72 °C for 15 seconds) and Group BC (n:10) did not receive any treatment and calves in this group were fed with pasteurised milk for 60 days. Blood GGT and total protein levels of calves used in the study were higher than 800 IU/l and 6 g/dl respectively. Body weight of all calves was measured just after birth and on day 60 of the study when calves were weaned. Feeding regimes were the same for all calves. Average daily weight gain (ADG) of calves was calculated by dividing the difference between birth and weaning weight by 60. Number of enteritis and pneumonia treatments were recorded. Treatment protocols were the same for both herds. Birth weights (±SEM) for AM, AC, BM and BC were 34.6±1.59; 34.6±1.68; 36.4±2.51 and 36.8±1.40 kg respectively. Weaning weights (±SEM) for AM, AC, BM and BC were 68.2±2.15; 65.9±1.89; 81,5±3.21; 72.8±2.38 kg, respectively. Weaning weights did not differ between AM and AC groups, but weaning weight of BM was significantly higher than BC ($P<0.05$). ADG (±SEM) for groups, AM, AC, BM and BC were 560±35, 522±25, 768±30 and 600±19 g, respectively. ADG of AM and AC was similar; however ADG of BM was significantly ($P<0.05$) higher than ADG of BC. Number of treatments for AM and AC groups was for enteritis 6 vs 5 and for pneumonia 3 vs 3 respectively. Calves from BM group received 6 enteritis and 5 pneumonia treatments however BC calves recieved 11 enteritis and 7 pneumonia treatments. We conclude that vitamin and trace element supplementation has beneficial effects on weight gain and health status of dairy calves fed pasteurised milk. However further studies evaluating blood vitamin and trace element levels in calves fed pasteurised milk are required.

Escherichia coli in industrial poultry production: aspects of transmission and disease development

J.P. Christensen[1], S.E. Pors[1], S. Papasolomontos[2], L.L. Poulsen[1], I. Thøfner[1], R.H. Olsen[1], H. Christensen[1] and M. Bisgaard[1]
[1]University of Copenhagen, Department of Veterinary Disease Biology, Stigboejlen 4, 1870 Frederiksberg C, Denmark, [2]VitaTrace Nutrition Ltd. (VITA), Propylaion 18, Strovolos Industrial Estate, 2033 Nicosia, Cyprus; jpch@sund.ku.dk

Escherichia coli is of major importance in commercial poultry production as the main cause of salpingitis and peritonitis in broiler parents and layers. In addition, first week mortality in young chicks and polyserositis in broilers continue to cause major losses to the industry. Chronic salpingitis, an often subclinical infection, has been suggested to represent a potential risk for vertical transmission and subsequent increased first week mortality. In one of our recent studies, four broiler parent flocks were followed during the whole production period by post mortem and bacteriological examination of randomly selected dead birds. Newly hatched chickens from each flock were swabbed in the cloaca and the bacterial flora analyzed. Causes of first week mortality were determined pathologically and bacteriologically. *E. coli* isolates were selected for pulsed-field-gel-electrophoresis and multi-locus-sequence-typing. *E. coli* was the main cause of both salpingitis in parents and first week mortality in broilers and *E. coli* dominated the bacterial flora of the cloaca of newly hatched chickens. Approximately one third of the mortality in the parents was due to salpingitis/peritonitis caused by *E. coli*. PFGE of *E. coli* showed identical band patterns in isolates from the three different sources (parents, hatcher & broilers) indicating a vertical transmission of *E. coli* from parent birds to chickens. We suggest that *E. coli* from salpingitis in broiler parents can be transmitted vertically and subsequently could spread in the hatcher. A single PFGE type dominated in one parent farm and this type was also found in the newly hatched chickens and as the aetiology of first week mortality. However, another study performed in our group clearly demonstrated that the use of a proper disinfection procedure has a significant impact on the reduction of cfu on eggshells indicating that disinfection of eggs is of major importance in reducing the frequency of *E. coli* caused first week mortality. Especially for *E. coli* the search for phylogenetic traits and genes, related to virulence and pathogenicity in salpingitis in egg-laying hens, has been described in several studies. However, suitable *in vivo* models enabling investigations of the impact of phylogenetics and the importance of specific genes for virulence *in vivo* are few and not directed towards infections of the oviduct. In this study, we report the development of an infection model able to differentiate between different *E. coli* isolates in relation to induced pathology and bacteriology.

Infections with Gram positive cocci in broiler breeders: significance and prevalence

I. Thøfner, L.L. Poulsen, R.H. Olsen, H. Christensen, M. Bisgaard and J.P. Christensen
University of Copenhagen, Faculty of Health and Medical Science, Department of Veterinary Disease Biology, Stigbøjlen 4, 1870 Frederiksberg C, Denmark; icnt@sund.ku.dk

In intensive poultry production systems good health and good management is crucial to obtain high levels of animal welfare and high production yields throughout the production cycle. In broiler breeders, decreased foot pad integrity mainly caused by poor litter conditions may subsequently result in an increase in mortality due to septicaemic infections, with sepsis, endocarditis and arthritis as the major manifestations, over time. Although the pathogenesis is not fully elucidated, the aetiology of these infections is often Gram positive (G+) cocci, such as *Staphylococcus* spp., *Enterococcus* spp. and *Streptococcus* spp. It is hypothesized that foot pad lesions serve as port of entry for systemic or localised bacterial infections. In a recent study we investigated the causes of the so-called normal mortality in four broiler breeder flocks from 20 to 60 weeks of age. Furthermore the individual foot pad health was recorded for each bird. Foot lesions were defined as presence of hyperkeratosis, ulcerations/necrosis or pododermatitis. Mortality caused by G+ cocci was low in young birds (20-29 weeks) but increased significantly during production, peaking in birds aged 40-49 weeks, overall resulting in approximately 13% of all the dead birds. The most frequently isolated G+ bacteria were *Staphylococcus aureus* and *Enterococcus faecalis*. Regardless the G+ aetiology, the observed lesions did not differ significantly, and most prevalent manifestations were arthritis, septicaemia and endocarditis. A significant fraction of these birds also displayed signs of systemic amyloidosis. During the observation period, we observed a strong correlation between foot pad health and age of dead birds with foot pad lesions increasing significantly from below 40% in young birds (20-29 weeks) to almost 80% in birds more than 50 weeks old. To further investigate these findings an experimental infection model using foot pads lesions as port of entry in old broiler breeders was established. Both *S. aureus* and *E. faecalis* strains where used as inoculum at different doses, by intradermal application in the central foot pad. Inoculation resulted in systemic lesions (sepsis, endocarditis and arthritis), corresponding to natural cases under field conditions, as well as injection site abscesses. Apparently, both strain, dose and time dependent bacteriological and pathological responses in relation to the experimental infection occur. This work is part of the EU-FP7 funded PROHEALTH project (grant n° 613574).

Effect of selection for growth rate on the resistance and tolerance of broilers to *Eimeria maxima*

P. Sakkas[1], I. Oikeh[1], R.A. Bailey[2], M.J. Nolan[3], D.P. Blake[3], A. Oxley[1], G. Lietz[1] and I. Kyriazakis[1]
[1]Newcastle University, AFRD, King's rd, NE1 7RU, Newcastle on Tyne, United Kingdom, [2]Aviagen Ltd, Newbridge, Edinburgh, EH28 8SZ, United Kingdom, [3]University of London, RVC, Department of Pathology and Pathogen Biology, Hawkshead Ln, Hatfield, AL9 7TA, United Kingdom; panagiotis.sakkas@ncl.ac.uk

We hypothesized that broilers selected for higher average daily gain (ADG) and lower feed conversion ratio (FCR) will have lower resistance to a coccidian challenge. 144 chicks of either a fast (F) or a slow growing (S) genotype were inoculated with 0, 2,500 (L), or 7,000 (H) sporulated *Eimeria maxima* oocysts at 13 days of age. Each treatment had 8 replicate pens with 6 birds/pen. ADG, feed intake (FI) and FCR post infection (pi) were calculated over the pre-patent (d1-4), acute (d5-8) and recovery phase (d9-12) of infection. To assess lesion score (LS), parasite replication (PR), and levels of zeaxanthin (z), lutein (l), a-tocopherol (at), and retinol (r) in plasma, birds were culled at d6 and d13pi. The relative values of the dependent variables of infected birds of the F and S genotype were calculated as the percentage difference of their respective controls. Genotype, dose, infection phase and their interaction were treated as factors for performance data and analysed with repeated measures mixed models, whilst single time point data were analysed with GLM. Average pen BW at d0pi was 478.9±4.5 and 371.4±2.9 (g) for F and S birds, respectively. Dose, phase, and their interaction affected ($P<0.0001$) ADG, FI and FCR, while genotype and phase interacted to impact FCR. Birds receiving the H and L dose showed reduced ADG (-13.7 vs -14.4; ±1.0), FI (-8.2 vs -9.8; ±0.9), and increased FCR (8.9 vs 7.0; ±1.1), effects being more pronounced during the acute phase. Infection impacted FCR to a higher degree in S as compared to F birds (10.4 vs 17.3; ±1.6) during the acute phase. PR and LS at d6pi were affected only by dose ($P<0.0001$), being similar among birds receiving the H and L dose. Lesions were not detected by d13pi. Infection reduced levels of z, l, r, and to ($P<0.0001$) at d6pi. By d13pi effects persisted for l ($P<0.05$), z and r ($P<0.01$), whilst r tended to be elevated in infected birds ($P<0.1$). At was affected by genotype ($P<0.05$) and tended to be affected by the interaction between genotype and dose ($P<0.1$); it was higher in F birds ($P<0.05$) and it was numerically higher for infected F than infected S birds. In conclusion, birds differing in their performance objectives showed similar resistance to infection. Contrary to our hypothesis, the impact of infection on FCR was greater in S than F birds at the acute phase of infection, and on at levels at the end of the recovery phase. This work is part of the EU FP7 funded PROHEALTH project (grant No 613574).

Control of dysbacteriosis in broilers by means of drinking water acidification

A. Cools[1], H. Slagter[1], C.D. Moor[1], A. Lauwaerts[1] and W. Merckx[2]
[1]Eastman Chemical Company, Pantserschipstraat 207, 9000 Ghent, Belgium, [2]ZTC Catholic University Leuven, Bijzondere weg 12, 3360 Lovenjoel, Belgium; ancools@eastman.com

Dysbacteriosis, a frequently occurring problem on broiler farms, is not only responsible for depressed performance but is also resulting in wet litter. Wet litter is one of the major causes of foot pad dermatitis, nowadays a major welfare issue. The aim of the present study was to investigate if performance of broilers as well as litter quality can be improved by supporting digestion and gut health by means of acidified drinking water. Two identical trials with 30 pens of 15 Ross 308 one day old male chicks per pen were set up. All animals were housed on wood shavings and fed a starter diet (crumble) for 14 days, followed by a grower and a finisher diet (both in pellet and during a 14 day period). In trial 1 half of the pens was offered regular drinking water (Control) whereas the other half was offered drinking water acidified with a blend of sodium buffered formic acid with propionic acid and copper sulphate (Protaq LF1). Trial 2 was set up similar to trial 1 but with a blend of sodium buffered formic acid with propionic acid and medium chain fatty acids (Protaq LF3) next to the Control. In both experiments pH of the acidified water was 4.2. On a pen level average daily gain (ADG), average daily feed intake (ADFI) and feed conversion rate (FCR) were measured. Litter scoring was done on a 0 to 3 scale (0 dry litter, 3 very wet litter) on days 28, 35 and 42. Statistics were done using RStudio and difference in performance between Control and treatment (Protaq LF1 or Protaq LF3) was investigated by means of a student's t-test. The effect of treatment on litter scoring was tested using a linear mixed model. Acidification of drinking water with Protaq LF1 resulted in increased ADG (55.9 ± 2.7 vs 58.4 ± 3.2 g; $P=0.026$) and reduced FCR (1.711 ± 0.054 vs 1.638 ± 0.060; $P=0.001$). Average litter score during the last 2 weeks was 2.37 with a significant reduction of 0.53 for the broilers drinking Protaq LF1 acidified water. When drinking water was acidified with Protaq LF3, ADG was not significantly different between Control and treatment but ADFI was reduced for the Protaq LF3 group (109.5 ± 2.5 vs 103.9 ± 7.7 g; $P=0.016$) resulting in an improved FCR (1.685 ± 0.077 vs 1.624 ± 0.090; $P=0.054$). Again, litter scoring during the last 2 weeks was on average 2.90 with a significant reduction of 1.17 for the Protaq LF3 supplemented broilers. Based on the results of these two experiments it can be concluded that acidification of drinking water can improve litter quality and performance of broilers. Further research on the impact of acidification on gut health and microbiota composition could give interesting insights in the mode of action.

Effect of genetic selection and physical activity on lameness and osteochondrosis prevalence in pigs

A. Boudon[1,2], M. Karhapää[3], H. Siljander-Rasi[3], N. Le Floc'h[1,2], E. Cantaloube[1,2] and M.C. Meunier-Salaün[1,2]

[1]Agrocampus Ouest, UMR 1348 PEGASE, Rue de St-Brieuc, 35000 Rennes, France, [2]INRA, UM 1348 PEGASE (Physiologie Environnement et Génétique pour l'Animal et le Système d'Elevage), Domaine de la Prise, 35590 Saint-Gilles, France, [3]Natural Resources Institute Finland, Green technology, PL 18, 01301 Vantaa, Finland; Anne.boudon@rennes.inra.fr

Locomotory disorders and more specifically lameness have been identified as one of the significant production diseases for growing and finishing pigs and sows. Lameness is a complex problem with multifactorial causes. Among these causes, osteochondrosis has a very high prevalence in all common pig breeds. Osteochondrosis is a local failure of epiphysis endochondral ossification that can be responsible, in its more severe form, of cracks at the level of joint cartilage. However, the proportion of lameness that can be linked to osteochondrosis is difficult to evaluate and still unknown. The PROHEALTH project aims at evaluating the influence of genetic selection on productive traits on the prevalence of leg disorders and to develop a methodology to assess lameness and osteochondrosis. For this purpose, 3 experiments aimed at measuring the prevalence of osteochondrosis in several populations of pigs. The tested pig populations included two divergent lines of Large-White selected for a feed efficiency trait (high or low residual feed intake) and two lines of Landrace selected for either their high fertility performance or their high growth performance. The Large-White populations were submitted to different constraints on the physical activity. These experiments also allowed identifying sex effects as females, entire and castrated males were studied within similar populations. All these experiments showed that osteochondrosis is very common in femur and humerus joints. In Landrace pigs, only 11% of the examined joints (539) were discovered as normal and 89% of joints had some signs of osteochondrosis. Within each breed, Large-White or Landrace, the osteochondrosis prevalence was not different between the compared lines but an effect the sex was observed. Boars were more susceptible for osteochondrosis than gilts. A question arises about the relevance of blood bio-markers of cartilage synthesis or turnover for easy and early diagnosis of osteochondrosis. The correlation between the serum concentrations of these bio-markers and the osteochondrosis scores remained low even if the reproducibility of these analyses during the animals' life were quite high.

Impact of poor hygiene on health and performance of pigs divergently selected for feed efficiency

A. Chatelet[1], E. Merlot[1], F. Gondret[1], H. Gilbert[2] and N. Le Floc'h[1]
[1]INRA, UMR PEGASE, 35590 Saint-Gilles, France, [2]INRA, UMR GenPhySE, 31326 Castanet-Tolosan, France; alexandra.chatelet@rennes.inra.fr

Production diseases impair production efficiency and animal welfare. Pigs with improved productive traits are suspected to be more at risk to develop diseases because of a lower capacity to allocate their nutritional resources for health. The aim of this study was to assess health and performance of two pig lines divergently selected for feed efficiency and housed in good or poor hygiene environment. Poor hygiene is known to induce inflammatory disorders and reduce growth performance. Large-White male and female pigs (n=160) from 80 to 160 days of age were included in a 2×2 factorial design comparing 2 lines divergently selected for Residual Feed Intake (low RFI=more efficient and high RFI=less efficient) and housed in 2 hygienic conditions (clean (C) vs dirty (D), n=40/group). The experiment was divided in two successive periods: during the challenging period, from Week 0 (W0) to W6, pigs were either housed in C or D conditions; blood was collected at W0, W3 and W6. During the recovery period, from W6 to W12, all pigs were housed in clean conditions. Half of the pigs in each group were euthanized at W6 and the remaining pigs were euthanized at W12 to collect tissue and evaluate body composition. Throughout the experiment, pigs were individually penned and had free access to a standard growing diet. Body weight and signs of clinical diseases (cough, diarrhea, lameness) were weekly recorded. Blood was collected to assess indicators of inflammation (haptoglobin, blood formula) and metabolite concentrations. Prevalence of pleurisy and pneumonia at slaughter was greater for D than C pigs. Average daily gain (ADG) from W0 to W6 was lower in D than C pigs, and this reduction was greater for the high RFI line (-247 g/d) than for low RFI line (-107 g/d). At W3, D pigs exhibited greater blood haptoglobin and neutrophil contents than C pigs, showing that poor hygiene condition induced an inflammatory response. Disparities were observed between the two lines with higher haptoglobin in high RFI pigs and higher amount of neutrophils in low RFI pigs. From W6 to W12, ADG and health blood biomarkers did not differ between D and C pigs, suggesting that pigs had recovered. In conclusion, low RFI pigs were less affected by the environmental challenge, which disagrees with our initial hypothesis. Data to be obtained on metabolite concentrations and expression levels of genes related to immunity will allow determining if the line differences in the ability to cope with this sanitary challenge were related to differences in resource allocation, immune capacities or growth precocity. Research has received funding from the EU FP7 Prohealth project (no. 613574)

Molecular characterisation of idiopathic lumbar kyphosis in pigs

A. Clark[1], I. Kyriazakis[1], C.R.G. Lewis[2], R. Farquhar[3] and G. Lietz[1]
[1]School of Agriculture, Food and Rural Development, Newcastle University, Newcastle Upon Tyne, NE1 7RU, United Kingdom, [2]Genus PIC, 100 Bluegrass Commons Blvd, Suite 2200, Hendersonville, TN, USA, [3]BQP, 1 New Street, Stradbroke, Eye, Suffolk, IP21 5JJ, United Kingdom; a.clark@newcastle.ac.uk

A humpy-backed syndrome of pigs has persisted in the British pork industry and causes of the deformity have been difficult to identify. The disease presents challenges in regards to handling the carcass and is suspected to slow down growth rate. There is no clear evidence of the biological mechanisms by which kyphosis is induced. Through collecting tissue samples from affected and healthy pigs over 3 age groups, this study aimed to identify molecular mechanisms induced by kyphosis. A range of tissue samples such as serum, liver, kidney, small intestine, bone and vertebral cartilage were dissected from kyphotic and control pigs at pre-weaning (2 weeks), weaning (5 weeks) and post-weaning (13 weeks). RNA was extracted from tissue samples using the RNeasy lipid tissue mini-kit (Qiagen) and cDNA was synthesised using the Transcriptor first strand cDNA synthesis kit (Roche). Expression levels of BMP7, a marker of bone mineralisation activity, were quantified by qPCR using SYBR green assays (DNA Essential Green Master mix, Roche) and expression levels normalised using the housekeeper gene RPL37. Preliminary results from qPCR analysis indicated a decrease in BMP7 expression in the vertebral cartilage of pre-weaning kyphotic pigs compared to age matched control pigs. Interestingly, BMP7 expression reduced from pre-weaning to weaning in healthy pigs ($P<0.05$) but remained constant for kyphotic pigs in both age groups. The array suggests kyphotic pre-weaners are not achieving sufficient cartilage mineralisation which would otherwise result in normal bone growth and development. Our initial results indicate reduced bone mineralisation in vertebral cartilage of pre-weaning kyphotic pigs. BMP7 expression was highest in healthy pigs at pre-weaning, most likely to facilitate bone growth in a rapidly growing period of development. Decreased cartilage mineralisation in kyphotic pre-weaners possibly facilitates widening of intervertebral disc space which conforms the spine into the characteristic hump-back. The results suggest that the highest risk of developing kyphosis occurs during the pre-weaning stage. This work was funded by the PROHEALTH project and Newcastle University.

Possible associations between environmental parameters and animal health in two fattening units

M. Klinkenberg[1], L. Vrielinck[2], D. Demeyer[2], T. Van Limbergen[1], E. Lorenzo[3], G. Montalvo[3], C. Piñeiro[3], J. Dewulf[1] and D. Maes[1]
[1]Ghent University, Faculty of Veterinary Medicine, Dept. of Reproduction, Obstetrics and, Herd Health, Belgium, [2]Danis, Group, NV, Vedanko, Belgium, [3]PigCHAMP, Pro, Europa, S.L., Spain; marlijn.klinkenberg@ugent.be

Environmental conditions in pig stables have an influence on pig health. Variations in temperature and drafts could lead to a higher prevalence of respiratory conditions. A longitudinal approach with multiple testing points could measure efficiently the effect of climatic and environmental conditions. Since this is time and resource consuming this is not often done. The objective of this study was to study the association between three environmental parameters and the number of diseased animals during one fattening period. Two fattening units were included with approximately 440 pigs each. Pigs were followed from the start of the fattening period until slaughter. Sensors were placed in the middle of both fattening units. The environmental parameters temperature (T, °C), relative humidity (RH, %) and CO_2 (ppm) were registered per hour. Measurements were conducted with General Alert™ Sensos. The number of diseased and treated animals were registered daily with a data capture system. The same animal could be scored multiple times over the whole period. Unit one was ventilated through a mechanical valve system, in unit two a natural ventilation system was used. The averages of the parameters during the day (7:00 am -19:00 pm) and during the night (19:00 pm - 7:00 am) were calculated for the two units separately. A two-sample T-test was performed to compare average temperature, CO_2 and RH in unit one and two (SPPS 22.0). Results Temperature, CO_2 and RH were normally distributed. In unit one average Tday was 22.48, Tnight was 22.26, CO_{2day} was 1,201.0, CO_{2night} was 1,382.7, RH_{day} was 65.47 and RH_{night} was 65.75. In unit two average T_{day} was 26.34, T_{night} was 26.37, CO_{2day} was 2,168.2, CO_{2night} was 2,138.4, RHday was 60.70 and RH_{night} was 59.40. Average temperature and CO_2 in unit 2 during the day and night were significantly higher, RH during the day and night was significantly lower. In unit one 175 animals obtained a score for respiration disorders, in unit two 535 animals. The differences in climate between the mechanically and naturally ventilated pig units seemed to have an influence on respiratory health in fattening pigs. Although the averages of the environmental parameters reflected a normal climate in a fattening unit, fluctuations over the day could have had an influence at the number of scored animals on a later time. At the moment, the relation between the climatic variability over the days and the health score is being studied. This work was conducted under the EU-funded PROHEALTH project.

What are the costs of poultry diseases: a review of nine production diseases

P.J. Jones[1], J. Niemi[2], R.B. Tranter[1] and R.M. Bennett[1]
[1]University of Reading, School of Agriculture, Policy and Development, P.O. Box 237, Earley Gate, University of Reading, Whiteknights, Reading, Berkshire, RG6 6AR, United Kingdom, [2]Natural Resources Institute Finland (Luke), Finland, Economics and society, Kampusranta 9, 60320 Seinäjoki, Finland; p.j.jones@reading.ac.uk

Diseases in poultry flocks can lead to substantial economic losses through reduced revenues, e.g. from lowered volume, or quality, of meat or eggs produced, and higher input costs. While this is widely understood, there is little consensus on the level of the economic losses resulting from individual production diseases. In addition, while the costs of prevention measures and treatments may be known, the economic savings they make are often not well understood. Consequently, large numbers of poultry producers may not be implementing economically optimal disease prevention and treatment measures. To explore the full economic impacts of poultry production diseases, an extensive survey of recent published studies was undertaken. From the literature review, data was collected on the incidence of nine key production diseases, the costs of these diseases when untreated, and the costs and benefits resulting from prevention or treatment measures. Data were collated from around 70 experimental, or field-scale, studies undertaken after 1990, based in regions with modern, commercial poultry production. In the reviewed studies, the most prevalent production diseases in broiler flocks are enteric, i.e. coccidiosis and clostridiosis, while in layers this is salpingoperitonitis. The costs of untreated diseases were found to vary markedly, and costs for individual diseases varied greatly with severity. Economic losses per bird in laying hens were found to be larger than for broilers, because the disease is impacting over a longer production period. Total economic losses from untreated keel bone damage averaged around €4 per laying hen, losses from infectious bronchitis reached €3.2 per hen and losses from salpingperitonitis could exceed €0.5 per paying hen. Losses more than €3 would, in most years, make the affected flock unprofitable. Among the broiler diseases, untreated clostridiosis incurred the greatest losses at around €1 per 2 kg broiler, while losses from untreated coccidiosis amounted to €0.21 per broiler. The review found that, in some cases, economic losses can be significantly reduced by prevention or treatment measures, but this capacity again varies markedly between diseases. For example, interventions for Salpingoperitonitis, ascites and clostridiosis can effectively eliminate output losses, but in the cases of coccidiosis and keel bone damage, studied interventions were much less effective.

Economic value of mitigating *Actinobacillus pleuropneumoniae* infections in pig fattening herds

A.H. Stygar[1,2], J.K. Niemi[3], C. Oliviero[4], T. Laurila[4] and M. Heinonen[4]
[1]*University of Copenhagen, Grønnegårdsvej 2, 1870 Frederiksberg C, Denmark,* [2]*MTT Agrifood Research Finland, Economic Research, Latokartanonkaari 9, 00790 Helsinki, Finland,* [3]*Natural Resources Institute Finland (Luke), Economics and society, Kampusranta 9, 60320 Seinäjoki, Finland,* [4]*University of Helsinki, Paroninkuja 20, 04920 Saarentaus, Finland; jarkko.niemi@luke.fi*

Actinobacillus pleuropneumoniae infections (APP) can cause severe economic losses in pig production. Swine producers can prevent the disease from occurring and spreading. However, to be profitable for the producer, the anticipated benefits of a mitigation policy should exceed its cost. In this study, a dynamic programming model and epidemic model (SIR) were developed, and policies for managing fattening pigs under the risk of APP infection were evaluated. The following disease mitigation options were considered: (1) cleaning including washing, drying and disinfection procedures; (2) cleaning and vaccination (with high, medium and low efficacy of vaccine); (3) cleaning and medication (antibiotics use). The results were calculated for five different levels of APP prevalence, where the disease can occur at ten levels of severity. The economic value of mitigation policy depended on the prevalence and severity of disease as well as on the efficiency of the implemented mitigation protocol. The results suggest that inefficient cleaning caused substantial economic losses which can reach up to €20.2 per pig space unit per year. The cleaning and vaccination policy was economically superior over the policy of only cleaning when the prevalence of disease was high (>0.3), there was a severe clinical disease and the medium or high efficacy vaccine was available. Moreover, even when vaccination costs were decreased the vaccination policy was not economically favored in situations with low disease prevalence among herds (0.1 and 0.3). In cases of severe disease, the cleaning and medication policy resulted in higher economic benefits than cleaning or cleaning and vaccination with low and medium efficacy vaccine. With a high prevalence (>0.3) and substantial decrease in the average daily gain (ADG), the joint application of cleaning and medication was economically less favorable than cleaning combined with the use of the high efficacy vaccine. Therefore, the availability of high efficacy vaccine could benefit farms facing the severe forms of APP and help to reduce the use of antibiotics. To avoid substantial economic losses, pig producers should not ignore cleaning procedures, which due to low efficacy of available vaccines and concerns regarding excessive use of antibiotics and antibiotic resistance in animal production should be the primary policy to mitigate APP. This work is part of the EU funded PROHEALTH project (grant No 613574).

Effect of a major gene on piglet response to co-infection with PRRSV and PCV2b

J.R. Dunkelberger[1], N.V.L. Serao[1,2], M. Niederwerder[3], M.A. Kerrigan[3], J.K. Lunney[4], R.R.R. Rowland[3] and J.C.M. Dekkers[1]
[1]Iowa State University, Ames, IA 50011, USA, [2]NC State University, Raleigh, NC 27695, USA, [3]Kansas State University, Manhattan, KS 66505, USA, [4]USDA, ARS, BARC, APDL, Beltsville, MD 20705, USA; jenelled@iastate.edu

Previously, a genetic marker (WUR) for a putative causative mutation in the GBP5 gene on chromosome 4 was associated with resistance to porcine reproductive and respiratory syndrome (PRRS), where the dominant B allele was associated with greater growth and lower serum viral load (VL) following PRRS virus (PRRSV) infection. Objectives were to estimate the effect of WUR and PRRS vaccination on co-infection with PRRSV and porcine circovirus type 2b (PCV2b) and to determine whether pigs with the favorable genotype respond better to vaccination. Two trials of 200 commercial nursery pigs were pre-selected based on WUR genotype (half AA/AB) and randomly sorted into two rooms. All pigs in one room received a modified live virus PRRS vaccine 28 days prior to co-infection with field strains of PRRSV and PCV2b and then followed for 42 days. PRRS VL post vaccination (Post Vx), post co-infection (Post Co-X), and PCV2b VL Post Co-X were calculated as the area under the curve of serum viremia from -28 to 0, 0 to 21, and 0 to 42 days post-infection (dpi), respectively. Average daily gain (ADG) was calculated as the regression of weight on dpi from -28 to 0 and 0 to 42 dpi for ADG Post Vx and Post Co-X, respectively. Vaccination resulted in slower growth ($P<0.001$) Post Vx and lower PRRS VL ($P<0.001$), higher PCV2b VL ($P<0.001$) but no detectable difference in ADG ($P=0.81$) Post Co-X. Compared to AA pigs, AB pigs had significantly lower PRRS VL upon first exposure to PRRS, whether by vaccination ($P=0.02$) or Co-X ($P<0.001$), and tended to have lower PRRS VL upon re-exposure [Vx pigs Post Co-X, ($P=0.06$)]. AB pigs also grew faster Post Vx ($P=0.02$), but not differently Post Co-X ($P=0.82$). For PCV2b VL, the effect of WUR ($P=0.09$) was greater for Vx pigs, for which AB pigs had significantly lower PCV2b VL ($P=0.01$) than AA pigs. However, the effect of WUR was not significantly different between vaccination groups for PRRS VL ($P=0.28$) or ADG ($P=0.51$) Post Co-X. Taken together, marker assisted selection based on WUR genotype is a promising strategy to select for improved response to PRRSV infection, but also co-infection with PCV2b and, perhaps, other pathogens. Numerically, the effect of WUR was greater upon first exposure to PRRSV, which is consistent with the role of GBP5 in innate immunity. WUR did have a significantly greater effect on PCV2b viremia following prior Vx for PRRS compared to no Vx, confirming the immunological interactions of PRRSV and PCV2b exposures. This research was supported by USDA-NIFA grants 2012-38420-19286 and 2013-68004-20362.

Reducing ammonia and the risk of disease in agriculture animals

G. Demko, W. Blakeley and P. Pearce
a better way for animals research foundation, research, 549 moose ridge, Athol, ID 83801, USA;
tofindhealth@ameritech.net

Independent field studies have demonstrated that a natural enzymatic mineral product improves digestion, nutrient absorption and the metabolic utilization of dietary protein. Importantly, this product reduces the amount of ammonia generated by digestive processes. This same natural liquid product has also been shown to reduce the number of potentially harmful microbial pathogens found in the digestive tract of agricultural animals. A formulation of food, trace minerals, ammonia and a natural liquid enzymatic amendment in water was placed in a laboratory-designed surrogate digestive tract of a chicken in a closed container. A stir plate with magnetic stir bar was used to simulate an animal's digestive tract motion. Connecting the container to a model Z-800XP ammonia monitor with a hose allowed for the recording of the gaseous ammonia concentration every minute. Two outside independent labs confirmed dramatic pathogen reduction of *Escherichia coli* and *Salmonella* species using this product. In accordance with accepted laboratory protocols, Anatek Labs confirms 100% removal of gaseous ammonia in the sealed container in nine of 10 samples. The average starting concentration was 116 ppm. The remaining test started at 232.2 ppm and reduced to 2.3 ppm. An organic nitrogen test in water using the EPA standard methodology was measured at 4, 6 and 14 days for ammonia, nitrites, nitrates and total Kjeldahl nitrogen. By day 14 all of the nitrites and nitrates were non-detectable. Ammonia decreased by 46.6%, TKN decreased by 74.7% and the production of organic nitrogen in the liquid increased over 200%. Michelson labs confirmed the pathogen reduction of *E. coli* 0157 by 99.8% (Log 2.73) and the reduction of *Salmonella* species by 99.3% (Log 2.18), thus indicating a significant reduction in pathogens. Nova lab, testing contaminated flood waters, confirmed *E. coli* ATCC 11229 decreased 96.533% (Log 1.46). Using this safe and natural enzymatic nutrient to eliminate elevated ammonia and significantly reduce the growth of pathogens can result in tremendous productivity and profitability benefits. This product requires minimal labor involvement and is safe, easy to implement, and economically feasible. Our original goals were to reduce ammonia and the risk of disease in animals and to demonstrate the effectiveness of this environmentally and animal safe natural enzymatic amendment. Continued research related to the application and implementation of this new technology for the existing and well-described problems in agriculture is indicated.

Identification of animal-based traits as indicators of production diseases in pigs

F. Loisel[1], S. Stravakakis[2], P. Sakkas[2], I. Kyriazakis[2], G. Stewart[2], N. Le Floc'h[1] and L. Montagne[1]
[1]INRA, Agrocampus Ouest, UMR1348 Pegase, 65 rue de Saint-Brieuc, 35000 Rennes, France,
[2]University of Newcastle, School of Agriculture, Food and Rural Development, Agriculture Building, NE1 7R, Newcastle upon Tyne, United Kingdom; lucile.montagne@agrocampus-ouest.fr

Production diseases induce loss of performance associated with the reduction in growth, feed efficiency and product quality, and increase in mortality and morbidity. This impacts on the profitability of a pig farm and goes against citizen acceptability of animal production. This study consisted of a systematic review of the published literature on production diseases affecting digestive, locomotory, and respiratory systems in pigs. It aimed to quantify the effect of these diseases on traits used to measure animal response. Data were extracted from 67 peer-reviewed publications selected from 2,339 records that resulted from an exhaustive online keyword search using a search engine. Traits were classified as productive traits (growth), behavioural, carcass (composition or dimensions), biochemical (concentration of a marker), and molecular traits for measures relative to DNA, RNA and protein expression. A meta-analysis based on mixed models was performed on traits assessed more than 5 times across studies, using the package metafor of the R software. A total of 524 unique traits were recorded 1 to 31 times in a variety of sample material including blood, muscle, articular cartilage, bone, or at the level of the animal for productive traits. No behavioural traits were recorded overall from the included experiments. 17 traits were measured more than five times across studies. The heterogeneity (I^2) within these traits and across studies was low (I^2=0%) for Crypt depth, Inflammatory biomarkers, and Cytokines such as Interleukine (IL) 6 and 8 and high for Feed conversion ratio, Melatonin and other cytokines, such as IL 1-beta and tumor necrosis factor alpha (I^2>60%). The traits mostly affected by the diseases were molecular and biochemical traits, specifically the inflammatory biomarkers Haptoglobin and Fibrinogen with effect sizes of 3.0 (Confidence interval (CI) 1.62-4.38) and 2.9 (CI 1.81-4.0), and cytokines such as IL 6 and 8, with effect sizes of 2.65 (CI 1.46-3.84) and 2.75 (CI 2.08-3.43), respectively. Average daily weight gain showed a summary effect size of -1.98 (CI -2.65 to -1.31) across studies. These traits can be considered as potential tools for the prognosis of production diseases or conversely to characterize healthy animals. This work is part of the EU-FP7 funded PROHEALTH project (grant n° 613574).

In vitro cytotoxicity and antiviral activity of plant extracts on avian infectious bronchitis virus

A. Šalomskas[1], R. Lelešius[1], A. Karpovaitė[1], R. Mickienė[2], T. Drevinskas[2], N. Tiso[2], O. Ragažinskienė[3], L. Kubilienė[4] and A. Maruška[2]

[1]Lithuanian university of health sciences, Department of infectious diseases, Tilžės g. 18, Kaunas, 47181, Lithuania, [2]Vytautas Magnus University, Faculty of Natural Sciences, Department of Biology, Vileikos g. 8-212, Kaunas, 44404, Lithuania, [3]Kaunas Botanical Garden of Vytautas Magnus University, Sector of Medicinal Plants, Žilibero g. 6, Kaunas, 46324, Lithuania, [4]Lithuanian University of Health Science, Faculty of Pharmacy, Sukilėlių pr. 13, Kaunas, 50166, Lithuania; algirdas.salomskas@lsmuni.lt

Avian infectious bronchitis (AIB) is an acute, highly contagious disease of major economic importance in commercial chicken flocks in Europe and Lithuania. Due to the low vaccination efficiency outbreaks of AIB virus often occurs in vaccinated flocks. One of the alternative methods for AIB prevention is the use of phytochemicals. The purpose of this work was the evaluation of cytotoxicity effect (CE) and screening for antiviral properties of medicinal plants and propolis extracts. Ethanol was used as control and 18 different extracts of medicinal plants and propolis were tested. Extracts were prepared using ethanol (40% vol.). Total amount of phenolic compounds, flavonoids and radical scavenging activity were determined spectrophotometrically. Composition of the phenolic compounds in the extracts was analysed chromatographically. CE was tested using Vero cells and Beaudette strain of AIB virus was used for antiviral properties testing. MTT assay was used for determination of CE. CE_{50} was calculated by linear regression analysis of the dose response curves. Inhibition of virus replication was evaluated by MTT assay and examination of the cells by light microscopy. Total amount of phenolic compounds varied in the extracts between 0.753-8.022 mg/ml, total amount of flavonoids between 0.041-2.486 mg/ml and radical scavenging activity between 0.326-13.47 mg/ml (expressed in rutin equivalents). The results of microscopy and MTT assay were correlated. Aqueous ethanol showed low CE while all plant and propolis extracts showed somewhat higher CE. Extract of *Agastache foeniculum* (Pursh) Kuntze showed the highest 6.32±0.13 $\log_2 CE_{50}$, while extracts of *Saturea montana* L., *Perilla frutescens* L. Britton., *Thymus vulgaris* L. and *Hyssopus officinalis* L. showed the lowest 2.75±0.11, 2.70±0.30, 2.98±0.09, and 2.97±0.10 $\log_2 CE_{50}$ respectively. The study of antiviral activity of extracts is in progress. The research showed that all extracts have various not high CE and they can be used fo rthe testing of antiviral properties. The research was granted by Research Council of Lithuania, project No. MIP-065/2015.

Molecular and functional heterogeneity of the early postnatal satellite cell population in the pig

K. Stange[1], C. Miersch[1], S. Hering[1], M. Kolisek[2] and M. Röntgen[1]

[1]Leibniz Institut for Farm Animal Biology (FBN), Muscle Biology & Growth, Wilhelm-Stahl-Allee 2, 18196 Dummerstorf, Germany, [2]Free University Berlin, Institute of Veterinary Physiology, Oertzenweg 19b, 14163 Berlin, Germany; stange@fbn-dummerstorf.de

During the pig postnatal life, hyperplastic and hypertrophic processes of skeletal muscle growth depend on activation, proliferation, differentiation and fusion of satellite cells (SCs) Therefore, its functional phenotype will greatly affect long-term growth performance and muscle health. In other species it has been demonstrated that SCs are a heterogeneous population. However this concept has never been explored in the pig. In this study, we isolated SCs from the longissimus and semimembranosus muscles of 4 day old piglets via digestion with trypsin (0.25%) and used a percoll gradient to separate two subpopulations (SP) of SCs. This SP were cultured over 3 passages (for 16 days) and characterized according to their growth kinetics and bioenergetic profile by using the xCELLigence system (ACEA Biosciences) and O_2-sensitive fluorescence sensors. Quantitative RT-PCR and flowcytometric analysis were performed to investigate the mRNA (Pax7, Myf5, MyoD, Desmin, and embryonic Myosin) and protein (Myogenin, Desmin and adult Myosin HC) expression of myogenic markers. Finally the ability to differentiate was investigated. 30% of isolated SCs constitute a fast adhering and fast proliferating (doubling time; DT: 16 h) subpopulation (SPF) while 70% showed considerable slower adhesion and proliferation (SPS, DT: 22 h). Between day 4 and day 8 of culture cell numbers increased approximately 5-fold in SPF cells compared with a 2.5-fold elevation of the cell number in SPS cells. Quantitative RT-PCR revealed increased RNA levels of the myogenic genes Pax7, MyoD, Desmin and embryonic Myosin in SPS cells whereas SPF cells expressed higher RNA levels of Myf5. Basal O_2 consumption rate and maximal respiration (an intrinsic property of mitochondria) were 30% and 36% higher in SPF than in SPS cells. Also, in the latter the ATP-synthase activity was actively down-regulated and reduced by 30% compared with SPF cells. Cells of both SP differentiated, but the fusion rates were higher (22 vs 15%) in SPF compared with SPS cells. In addition, a lower percentage of cells positive for Myogenin, Desmin and (adult) Myosin HC proteins were found in late (14 day old) SPS cultures. Our data clearly show the existence of intrinsically heterogeneous SC populations in the pig that could have different functions in postnatal muscle growth. Its better understanding can give implications to improve the growth performance, e.g. of low birth weight piglets. initial data show a reduced number of SPS cells in muscles of growth retarded piglets.

Antioxidant capacities of pigs were altered in a tissue-specific manner by poor hygiene conditions

K. Sierzant[1,2], E. Merlot[2], S. Tacher[2], N. Le Floc'h[2] and F. Gondret[2]
[1]*Wroclaw University of Environmental and Life Sciences, Faculty of Biology and Animal Science, 50137 Wroclaw, Poland,* [2]*INRA, UMR Pegase, 35590, France; florence.gondret@rennes.inra.fr*

Degradation of the environmental hygiene could alter growth rate and induce a systemic inflammatory response. Inflammation and oxidative stress are correlated pathways. Oxidative stress generally arises when antioxidant defenses are overhelmed by increased production of reactive oxygen species (ROS). Importantly, selection for residual feed intake (RFI) in growing pigs, a measure of feed efficiency, may also impact mitochondria ROS production. This study aimed at investigating systemic and tissue antioxidant capacities of pigs divergently selected for RFI and housed in poor or good hygiene conditions. During a 6-week challenge period, growing pigs of low (n=99) or high (n=73) RFI lines were housed in dirty (n=89) or in clean (n=83) conditions; half of the pigs were then killed to collect blood and tissues. The remaining pigs were transferred in a clean environment for an additional 8-week period (resilience), after what blood and tissues were collected. Poor hygiene conditions resulted in greater plasma levels of diacron reactive oxygen metabolite (dROM reflecting the amount of hydroperoxides), and a lower total antioxidant plasma capacity (ferric reducing ability [FRAP]). The increase in dROM to FRAP ratio observed in response to poor hygiene conditions was greater in the high RFI pigs than in the low RFI pigs. Poor hygiene conditions also activated antioxidant enzymes such as superoxide dismutase (SOD), catalase (CAT) and glutathione reductase (GSH-Rx) in perirenal adipose tissue, while SOD activity was decreased and CAT and GSH-Rx activities did not change in the liver of pigs raised in poor hygiene conditions. High RFI pigs exhibited higher activities of CAT and GSH-Rx in perirenal fat when compared with low RFI pigs, with no difference between lines in the liver. After the resilience period in clean conditions, there were no differences between pigs in plasma levels of oxidative and antioxidant markers. At that stage, antioxidant enzyme activities were higher in perirenal fat and liver of pigs having being challenged during early growth. In conclusion, poor hygiene conditions increased systemic oxidative stress and immediately activated antioxidant enzymes in adipose tissue, while liver responses seemed to be delayed. A greater susceptibility to systemic oxidative stress was also suggested for the less efficient (high RFI) pigs. Research has received funding from the EU FP7 program (PROHEALTH, grant agreement no. 613574). K. Sierzant received a grant from Wroclaw University (Faculty of Biology and Animal Science; program KNOW).

Identifying potential biomarkers to improve production in pigs and poultry

T. Giles[1], S. Hulme[1], P. Barrow[1], N. Le Floc'h[2], S. Schaeffer[2], A.M. Chaussé[2], P. Velge[2] and N. Foster[1]

[1]*University of Nottingham, School of Veterinary Medicine and Science, School of Veterinary Medicine and Science, University of Nottingham, LE12 5RD, United Kingdom,* [2]*INRA, Institut National de la Recherche Agronomique, Rennes, 35700 Rennes, France; timothy.giles@nottingham.ac.uk*

Work Package 5 of the Prohealth consortium aims to identify molecular markers that are associated with poor production in pigs and poultry. Microarrays are a powerful tool which will enable us to determine which genes are up- or down-regulated as a result of disease or environmental condition. Application of software analysis packages such as GeneSpring will allow us to link these genes to physiological or immunological pathways and help us identify genes or sets of genes which have predictive value in identifying at risk animals. As part of an EU wide consortium, we have access to samples from a variety of countries including Belgium, Spain, France and the Republic of Ireland. Agilent 4x44K microarrays will be used to analyse the changes in gene expression from animals reared in different commercial and experimental farms. Preliminary work has focused on data obtained from an experimental design performed at INRA (France) on Large-White pigs housed in poor or high hygiene conditions and exhibiting clear differences in growth performance and plasma immune status. RNA from tissue samples preserved in RNAlater have been hybridised on microarrays at the University of Nottingham (UK). Initial results from arrays have been compared with results obtained using a Biomark high-throughput RT-PCR device (Fluidigm) at INRA. Preliminary data indicates that the two methods show similar results. Initially, only the immune-related genes were analysed by microarray, since prior to microarray analysis, the Biomark analysis was used to assess expression of 96 immune-related genes in three different tissues (mesenteric lymph nodes, tracheobronchial lymph nodes and Peyer's patches) from pigs bred in poor or high hygiene conditions. Array results indicated that over 30 immune-related genes were differentially expressed in pigs raised on high hygiene farms compared to those raised on low hygiene farms. These results are supported by data obtained by INRA where 26 genes had greater than a twofold change in expression. Genes including TNFa, IL23R and STAT3, which are associated with the Th17 axis and which represent a pro-inflammatory subset of T cells, were up-regulated in pigs reared on low hygiene farms. Ingenuity Pathway Analysis will be used to recognise specific gene pathways and identify potential biomarkers. Further work will be carried out which will study specific diseases of importance in the pig and poultry industry.

Interaction between metabolism, immune function and uterine health in postpartum dairy cows

G. Opsomer, O. Bogado Pascottini and M. Hostens

Department of Reproduction, Obstetrics and Herd Health, Faculty of Veterinary Medicine, Ghent University, Salisburylaan 133, 9820 Merelbeke, Belgium; geert.opsomer@ugent.be

The multiple number of papers discussing the definitions of metritis and endometritis illustrates the continuous debate on this topic. More recent definitions are based on clinical signs to better match clinical findings with experimental studies. Since several years, subclinical endometritis (SCE) has been added to the list of postpartum uterine anomalies in cattle, defined as the presence of an elevated number of polymorphonuclear cells (PMNs) in the uterine lumen impairing pregnancy outcome at an eventual insemination. Studies in several countries have led to variable results concerning both prevalence as well as impact of this subclinical disease. Recently, we created an innovative device to sample cows during insemination: the cytotape (CT). The CT allows to assess the incidence of SCE at insemination and directly determines the effect of the elevated number of PMNs on the pregnancy outcome. We have assessed preliminary results of 1,947 AI-CT samples performed in nulliparous heifers and lactating dairy cows by one single inseminator. An insemination was considered successful when pregnancy was confirmed by rectal palpation at least 45 d post-AI, and not successful when diagnosed not pregnant or followed by a subsequent insemination. Using an arbitrary cut-off point of 3% of PMNs, the SCE prevalence in heifers was 4.7% (n=24) while in cows it was 13.85% (n=329). The overall conception rate in heifers was 61.19%. In SCE positive heifers (n=19), the conception rate was 31.57%, versus 62.5% (P<0.01) in their negative counterparts (n=432). In cows, the overall conception rate was 43.58%. In SCE positive cows (n=217), the conception rate was 27.18% versus 46.36% (P<0.01) in SCE negative cows (n=1279). In conclusion, satisfactory endometrial cytology samples were harvested during AI using the CT technique. Subclinical endometritis diagnosed during AI seems to decrease the risk for conception. A more extensive analysis of the data is needed to assess the importance of diagnosing SCE during an insemination, taking into account other covariates that affect fertility. This analysis will allow us to set a threshold for the percentage of PMNs in a CT-sample at AI, associated with the pregnancy outcome of that insemination. An even more intriguing question is, why so many dairy cows still suffer from SCE at insemination. Several research papers claim that at that time postpartum bacterial infections are no longer the reason to attract PMNs to the endometrium. Therefore, we currently hypothesize 'metinflammation' might be the underlying cause of SCE, with high circulating levels of non-esterified fatty acids as an important contributing factor.

Relationships of uterine health with metabolism in dairy cows with different dry period lengths

J. Chen[1], N.M. Soede[1], G.J. Remmelink[2], R.M. Bruckmaier[3], B. Kemp[1] and A.T.M. Van Knegsel[1]
[1]Wageningen University, Adaptation Physiology Group, Department of Animal Sciences, P.O. Box 338, 6700 AH Wageningen, the Netherlands, [2]Wageningen University and Research Centre, Livestock Research, P.O. Box 338, 6700 AH Wageningen, the Netherlands, [3]University of Bern, Veterinary Physiology, Vetsuisse Faculty, Bremgartenstrasse 109a, 3001 Bern, Switzerland; juncai.chen@wur.nl

The recovery of a healthy uterine environment after parturition is a key factor for reproductive success in dairy cows. It is unclear how uterine health relates with milk yield and metabolic status in dairy cows with a shortened or omitted dry period. Therefore, the objective of the current study was to evaluate relationships of uterine health with milk yield, and metabolic status in dairy cows with different dry period lengths in the second year after implementation of dry period length treatment. For this study, Holstein-Friesian dairy cows (n=130) were assigned randomly to 1 of 3 dry period lengths (0-, 30-, or 60-d) for 2 consecutive years. A vaginal discharge score (VDS) was taken in wk 2 and wk 3 after calving to evaluate uterine health status and cows were classified as having a healthy uterine environment (HU, VDS=0 or 1 in both wk 2 and 3), a recovering uterine environment (RU, VDS=2 or 3 in wk 2 and VDS=0 or 1 in wk 3), or a non-recovering uterine environment (NRU, VDS=2 or 3 in wk 3). Cows were monitored for milk yield and DMI from calving to wk 3 after calving. Blood was sampled weekly from calving to wk 3 after calving. Vaginal discharge score was not affected by dry period length. Independent of dry period length, NRU cows had lower milk yield (*P<0.01*) and lower DMI (*P<0.01*) in the first 3 wk after calving compared with HU or RU cows. In the first 3 wk after calving, RU cows had lower plasma glucose (*P<0.01*) and insulin (*P=0.03*) concentrations compared with NRU or HU cows. RU cows tended to have a lower plasma urea concentration (*P=0.05*) compared with HU cows. In conclusion, dry period length had no effect on the recovery of a healthy uterine environment in dairy cows. Independent of dry period length, cows with a non-recovering uterine environment had a decreased DMI and milk yield. Cow with a healthy uterine environment had a high milk yield and also a better metabolic status in early lactation, as indicated by greater plasma glucose and insulin concentrations.

Automatically recorded body condition scores: patterns and associations with fertility
U. Emanuelson[1], S. Granz[2] and C. Hallén Sandgren[3]
[1]Swedish University of Agricultural Sciences, Dep't Clinical Sciences, P.O. Box 7054, 75007 Uppsala, Sweden, [2]DeLaval Services GmbH, Wilhelm-Bergner-Str. 3, 21509 Glinde, Germany, [3]DeLaval International, P.O. Box 39, 147 21 Tumba, Sweden; ulf.emanuelson@slu.se

Transition cow management is important for both production and reproductive efficiency. Body condition scoring (BCS) of dairy cows is recognized as being an important factor in dairy cattle management, especially for the transition cow. The BCS at calving, the lowest BCS (nadir), and the amount of BCS-loss post-calving are associated with milk production, reproduction, and health. The aim of the present study was to derive BCS-patterns, based on BCS recorded on a scale from 1 to 5 in an automatic system with a continuously running 3D camera linked to a RFID system (DeLaval BCS camera), and their associations with fertility indicators. The study was based on weekly averages of the BCS-recordings from four herds in three countries, with a period of BCS-recordings ranging from 232 to 679 days. Two of the herds had pure Holstein Friesian (HF) cows, one Simmental and one 75% Norwegian Red (NRF) and 25% HF crosses. The median number of cows recorded any day in the herds varied between 55 and 528, and the average daily milk yield in the herds varied between 27.3 and 29.2 kg. The BCS-patterns calculated were BCS at the first or second week after calving (BCSinit), the lowest BCS (BCSnadir), week in milk at BCS nadir (BCSnadirw) and total loss of BCS at nadir (BCSloss), while days from calving to first AI (CFI) was used as the fertility indicator. Associations between the BCS-patterns and CFI were assessed with survival analysis models, where cows without any AI were censored at the last BCS record. The models also included parity (1, 2, 3+) and season of calving as fixed effects and herd as a random shared frailty effect. Median BCSinit was 3.37 (inter-quartile range (IQR) 3.09; 3.62) and corresponding figures for BCSnadir, BCSnadirw and BCSloss were 3.07 (2.76; 3.36), 4 (2; 6) and -0.22 (-0.11; -0.35), respectively. There was a large between-farm variation, especially for BCSloss where the medians were -0.14, -0.18, -0.23 and -0.30, with the lowest loss in the NRF-herd and highest in the HF-herds. Median CFI (IQR) was 77 days (57; 104), with medians for the four herds 52, 69, 82 and 83 days, where the longest were for the HF-herds. BCSinit and BCSnadir were significantly associated with CFI, where a higher BCS at calving and at nadir were associated with shorter CFI, while neither BCSnadirw nor BCSloss were significantly associated with CFI. The automatic recording of BCS was useful in deriving BCS-patterns, which can be used for herd management purposes. Also, BCS at calving and at nadir can be an important predictor for CFI in these herds.

Interaction between conception, mastitis and subclinical ketosis in dairy cows

A. Albaaj, G. Foucras and D. Raboisson
National School of Veterinary, 23 chemin des Capelles, BP 87614, 31076 Toulouse Cedex 3,
France; a.albaaj@envt.fr

The success rate of conception is decreasing year after year worldwide. Mastitis has been associated with deteriorated reproduction performances and subclinical ketosis (SCK) was also reported as a risk factor of decreased conception. This work provides an attempt to describe how SCK may modulate the reported association between mastitis and conception in dairy cows. French data from Milk Control Program and data on artificial insemination (AI) were included for 5 years (2008-2012). Mastitis was evaluated through the high (H) or low (L) level of somatic cell counts (SCC) before and after AI and transformed into 4 classes (LL, and LH, HL, HH) relative to various thresholds. SCK was defined through milk fat and protein content or their ratio before and after AI. Test days 0-40 or 40-80 days before and after AI were considered alternatively. Conception was introduced in models as a binary trait and was explained by the udder health, SCK and their interaction. All statistical models were adjusted by days in milk, milk yield and parity and herd was kept as random effect. Conception was reduced by 10, 15, 20 and 26% for cows with high SCC after AI (LH and HH classes) when SCC thresholds were 100,000, 200,000, 400,000 and 800,000 cells/ml, respectively. Applying the same analysis only on the subpopulation with SCK showed a lower relative risk (RR) of conception in cases of mastitis. The difference could be as high as 12 percentage points. Including the interaction term SCC×SCK clearly showed that SCK modulated the association between SCC classes and conception. The reduction in conception observed for LH with SCK compared to LL without any SCK was up to 25%. The present study confirms the previous findings about the negative association between mastitis around or after AI and a decreased rate of conception. It also highlights how SCK modulates the above-mentioned relationship by increasing the strength of the interaction between mastitis and conception. The present work also supports the theory that a local inflammation may affect the entire body response and alters the functions of other organs like the reproductive tract.

Lymphoid aggregates are associated with reduced placental mass and embryonic loss in dairy cows

M.C. Lucy, T.J. Evans and S.E. Poock

Univeristy of Missouri, Columbia, 65211, USA; lucym@missouri.edu

Lymphoid aggregates (also known as lymphocytic foci) form within the bovine endometrium after antigenic challenge. Their presence in the pregnant uterus may represent cytological evidence for an early postpartum uterine infection and could explain greater embryonic loss in dairy cows with early postpartum uterine disease. The objectives were to characterize the size and location of the aggregates in the pregnant uterus; determine their composition by using immunohistochemistry; and associate their presence with uterine tissue morphology, development of the pregnancy, and embryonic loss. Pregnant cows (n=43) were slaughtered on d 28, 35, or 42 of pregnancy. Uterine tissue was collected and processed for histological and immunohistochemical analyses. The number of small (<100 micron diameter), intermediate (100 to 250 micron diameter) and large (>250 micron diameter) lymphoid aggregates was counted. The number of cows averaging 0, 0.1 to 1, 1.1 to 2, and greater than 2 aggregates per section (small, intermediate, and large; combined) was 7 (16%), 14 (33%), 11 (26%) and 11 (26%), respectively. The average number of lymphoid aggregates found in the histological sections was greater in cows with evidence of uterine infection postpartum ($P<0.05$). Lymphoid aggregates were distributed within the caruncular and the intercaruncular tissue and were comprised of a core of CD3 positive cells (T cells) surrounding CD79 positive cells (B cells). The number of lymphoid aggregates was correlated with the number of inflammatory cells in the stratum compactum ($r^2=0.34$; $P<0.001$) and the amount of periglandular fibrosis in the endometrium ($r^2=0.33$; $P<0.001$). Cows with a high aggregate count had lesser placental weight on day 35 ($P<0.05$) and 42 ($P<0.01$) of pregnancy. There was no effect of aggregate count on placental weight on day 28. Two cows with embryonic loss were in the highest quartile for lymphoid aggregate count. In conclusion, cows with a large number of lymphoid aggregates in the uterine endometrium had more inflammation and fibrosis in the pregnant uterus and reduced placental weight on d 35 and 42 of pregnancy. The number of aggregates in pregnant cows was associated with early postpartum uterine disease. Whether the aggregates themselves are inhibitory to pregnancy development or the aggregates are associated with an inhibitory bacteriological, morphological or biochemical imprint left by early postpartum uterine disease will need to be investigated.

Hepatic mineral concentrations and health status in bovine fetuses

R.J. Van Saun

Pennsylvania State University, Veterinary & Biomedical Sciences, 115 Henning Building, 16802,
USA; rjv10@psu.edu

Fetal abortion and stillbirth are significant pregnancy wastage events contributing to low reproductive efficiency in dairy and beef cattle. The study objective was to determine if hepatic trace mineral concentration differences were present among abattoir, aborted and stillborn beef and dairy calves in suggesting a potential role for mineral nutrition in perinatal calf losses. Hepatic mineral concentrations (n=318) were retrospectively compared across aborted (n=71) and stillborn (n=62) calves. A population of fetal livers were collected from an abattoir (n=185) were used as 'healthy' control comparisons. All liver mineral concentrations were determined by the same university laboratory by inductively coupled plasma spectroscopy (ICP/MS) methods. Mineral concentrations were determined on a wet weight (WW) basis and converted to dry weight (DW) basis using determined liver dry matter content. Measured minerals included calcium (Ca), cobalt (Co), iron (Fe), magnesium (Mg), manganese (Mn), selenium (Se) and zinc (Zn). Abortion and stillborn submissions were categorized based on laboratory diagnosis as either dystocia, infectious or idiopathic. Population source (abattoir, abortion, stillborn), gender, age, breed and other descriptive information were collected. Analysis of variance (ANOVA) models were used to determine main effects of source, disease status, breed (dairy, beef) and all interactions on hepatic mineral concentration. Breed was not equally distributed among categories and significantly influenced all mineral concentrations, except Mn, thus was used as a covariate in all models. Beef calves independent of disease status had higher Mo, Fe, Co and Ca hepatic concentrations compared to dairy calves, whereas all other minerals were higher in dairy calves. Disease category influenced Cu (P=0.0006), Co, Mg (P<0.0001), Mo (P=0.01) and Zn (P=0.0036). No source by disease category interactions were found. Source by breed interaction influenced Ca (P=0.0002), Cu (P=0.0012), Co (P<0.0001), and Mg (P=0.009). Infectious or idiopathic causes of abortion or stillbirth had lower Cu, Mg and Zn and higher Mo concentrations compared to abattoir samples and dystocia stillbirths. Hepatic mineral concentrations were not different between abattoir and dystocia calves. These data are similar to other reports indicating lower hepatic mineral concentrations in abortion cases and add further support to suggest infectious and idiopathic abortion or stillborn may have underlying nutritional deficits. Breed effects are most likely a function of differences in mineral intake and source with potential inhibitors. Further study to validate these associations and better define specific hepatic mineral concentration diagnostic criteria are needed.

Searching for an effective BVD eradication program for the Netherlands

D.A. Kalkowska, M. Werkman, A.A. De Koeijer and W.H.M. Van Der Poel
Central Veterinary Institute of Wageningen UR, Bacteriology and Epidemiology, Houtribweg 39,
8221 RA Lelystad, the Netherlands; dominika.kalkowska@wur.nl

Bovine viral diarrhoea (BVD) is an infectious disease generally most severe in young stock. Infections in bovines can be divided in two types: transient infection (TI) and persistent infection (PI). A TI normally results in relatively mild symptoms and recovery after around 10 days. In contrary, PI animals remain extremely infectious during their full life span. These animals have a very high mortality during the early days of their lives. Up to 70% of PI animals do not reach the production age (2 years). The surviving PI animals will, if they give birth, create new PI calves. BVD infection in susceptible pregnant dams gives a high probability of abortion (up to 80%) and birth of PI calves, depending on the state of gestation at infection. Consequently, the presence of a PI-animal results in substantial production losses for individual farmers (estimated at €30 to €60 per cow). BVD is endemic in the Netherlands and one of its most significant reproductive disorders in cattle. Approximately 1-2% of cattle are PIs. Since many European countries are in the process of BVD-eradication, the export potential of the Netherlands is decreasing. In combination with the direct economic impact, eradication of BVD has become an important for the Dutch cattle industry. In the absence of a European eradication strategy, we look for t a cost-effective strategy, with as few imposed measures as possible.. To investigate the most effective control strategy, we developed a stochastic model for BVD transmission and eradication. In the model, the animals are classified as maternal immune (M), susceptible (S), TI, PI and recovered (R). Within herd transmission is performed by the Gillespie algorithm. We included all Dutch farms distributed over the following herd types: dairy, young stock raising, veal calves, bulls, other beef, suckling cows, cattle traders, cattle collection centres and small cattle holdings. We categorised age structure that covers production status for each herd type individually. Transmission between farms can occur through live animal movements. Moreover, the model includes the current certification program for BVD, which is based on ear biopsies, serology and/or bulk milk (BM) screening. In the model, we determine the key elements influencing the efficacy of a control strategy, based on specific risk factors (such as veal calve import), restriction of live animal movements and the impact of non-dairy farm types on national prevalence. Furthermore, we estimate the time until the disease free status is achieved and economical costs of eradication.

Relationship between ovulation rate in sows and litter characteristics at birth

C.L.A. Da Silva[1], D.B. De Koning[1], B.F.A. Laurenssen[1], H.A. Mulder[2], E.F. Knol[3], B. Kemp[1] and N.M. Soede[1]
[1]Wageningen University, Adaptation Physiology Group, De Elst, P.O. Box 338, 6700 AH, Wageningen, the Netherlands, [2]Wageningen University, Animal Breeding and Genomics Centre, Droevendaalsesteeg 1, P.O. Box 338, 6700 AH, Wageningen, the Netherlands, [3]Topigs Norsvin Research Center B.V., Helvoirt, P.O. Box 86, 5268 ZH, Beuningen, the Netherlands; carolina.lima@wur.nl

Modern hybrid sows have a high ovulation rate (OR). A high OR has been linearly related with decreased uterine implantation length and placental length at day 35 of pregnancy, which could inhibit foetal growth during further pregnancy and result in decreased piglet birth weight and increased within litter birth weight variation. Thus, we investigated the relationship between OR and litter characteristics at birth. Multiparous (parities 2-9) crossbred sows (Yorkshire × Landrace, n=109) were submitted to transrectal real time B-mode ultrasonography at day 24±2.6 of pregnancy. The number of corpora lutea on the left and right ovaries indicated OR. At farrowing, litter size (LS, born alive + stillborn), average piglet birth weight (BW) and the standard deviation of piglet birth weight (SDBW) within litters were assessed. The associations of OR with litter characteristics were assessed in statistical models also taking into account LS. The average OR was 25.2±3.8 (range 16 to 33), LS was 17.7±3.1 piglets, BW was 1,293±188 g and SDBW was 306±76 g. OR had a negative curvilinear relation ($P<0.05$) with LS (LS = 2.06±0.84 × OR – 0.04±0.02 × OR^2), with a maximum of 18.2±0.54 piglets at 25 ovulations. BW had a positive curvilinear ($P<0.05$) relation with OR (BW=-117.8±47.3 × OR + 2.25±0.94 × OR^2 + C. The value of C depended on LS class: 2,886.5±634.4 (LS 8-16; n=39), 2,799.4±634.2 (LS 17-19; n=40) or 2,684.9±593.6 (LS 20-26; n=30). Thus, at 26 ovulations, a minimum BW was observed of 1,346±31 g (LS 8-16), 1,259±32 g (LS 17-19) and 1,144±33 g (LS 20-26), respectively. SDBW was not significantly related with OR ($P\geq0.05$). In conclusion, sows with an average OR of 25-26 have the highest average LS and the lowest average piglet BW. The lower LS and higher BW observed in sows with more than 25-26 ovulations might be explained by a higher incidence of embryonic mortality before uterine implantation resulting from reduced early embryonic quality. The early embryonic mortality would increase the uterine space resulting in better placental development, and with a better placental development further foetal development would be favoured, increasing BW. Since the highest LS and lowest piglet BW is observed at the average OR of 25-26, this suggests that focus of selection should be on an increase in uterine capacity, to increase piglet BW in these sows.

Lactational oestrus in group housed lactating sows

B.F.A. Laurenssen, J.E.M. Strous, S.E. Van Nieuwamerongen, J.E. Bolhuis, C.M.C. Van Der Peet-Schwering and N.M. Soede

Wageningen University, Adaptation Physiology Group, De Elst 1, 6700 AH, the Netherlands; bjorge.laurenssen@wur.nl

One way to improve post-weaning piglet welfare, is to prolong the lactation period. However, as sows are normally anoestrous during lactation, a prolonged lactation will result in a reduction in the number of piglets produced per sow per year. It is possible to induce a fertile oestrus during lactation using an intermittent suckling strategy (IS). This is a management strategy in which the daily suckling frequency is reduced by limiting the time sows and piglets spend together. This study evaluated effects of IS in the 5th week of a 6-week (batch 1-4) or 9-week (batch 5-8) lactation period on reproductive performance of group-housed lactating sows. Per batch, 4-5 multiparous sows were housed in a multi-suckling system. IS started after four weeks of lactation (= IS-Day 0) and sows were separated from their piglets 10 h/day for 7 days. During separation, sows were moved to an adjacent IS-area, where a boar was present in a boar pen. After week 5, sows had voluntary access to the IS area 24 h/day. In this area, the back-pressure test was performed twice a day in presence of the boar for oestrus detection. At IS-Day 0 and IS-Day 5, transrectal ultrasound was used to assess ovarian status and to measure the 5 largest follicles per ovary. A pregnancy check was performed 4 weeks after insemination. In total, 29 out of 39 sows (74%) came in oestrus at 5.5±1.4 (3-9) days after onset of IS and the majority of those came in oestrus at IS-Day 5 (48%). One additional sow came in oestrus in week 7 of lactation. In total 28 of the 29 sows that showed oestrus during IS ovulated and 26 of these 28 sows (93%) were pregnant at day 28 after insemination. Subsequent litter size was 17.4±3.4 (based on 20 litters so far). Sows that came in oestrus during IS had a larger follicle size at IS-Day 0 (3.6±0.4 vs 3.2±0.4 mm, $P=0.01$) and at IS-Day 5 (6.2±0.8 vs 5.3±0.9 mm, $P=0.01$) than sows that did not show oestrus. They also had thicker backfat at IS-Day 0 (14.2±2.9 vs 11.5±3.0 mm, $P=0.01$); 90% of the 21 sows with a backfat >12.5 mm came in oestrus compared to 50% of the 18 sows with lower backfat. There was no difference in sow parity (3.2±1.6), sow weight at IS-Day 0 (222±30) or litter size at IS-Day 0 (11.6±1.7) between sows that did and did not come in oestrus during IS. In conclusion, IS can be a good method to induce lactational oestrus and pregnancy in group-housed lactating sows, resulting in good litter size. Sows should be in a good body condition at onset of IS to increase the chance of oestrus induction. These findings are a promising step for the further development of systems with longer lactation periods while safeguarding the number of piglets produced per sow per year.

Influence of fiber and amino acids on farrowing process, sow health and piglet vitality

X. Benthem De Grave, P. Van Der Aar and F. Molist
Schothorst Feed Research, Meerkoetenweg 26, 8218 NA Lelystad, the Netherlands;
xbenthemdegrave@schothorst.nl

Increasing litter size emphasized issues related to intense nutritional requirements of the lactating sow and to health and welfare related concerns like piglet vitality and post-partum dysgalactia syndrome (PDS). Questions remain about the need for increased supply of balanced amino acids (AA), or about the role of dietary fiber, either fermentable (fCHO) or inert (iCHO) carbohydrates (fecal digestibility), to improve farrowing process and growth of the offspring. Hundred fifty sows entering farrowing room were allocated to one of 6 diets until weaning, in a factorial arrangement of 2 AA levels (basal 6.7 g SID Lys/kg vs +40%) and 3 dietary fiber types (basal, +40% fCHO, +60% iCHO). Performance of sows and piglets was recorded until day of return to estrus. Farrowing process was studied on 12 sows per treatment, in addition to stress, PDS and faecal scores. Piglet birth time, individual weight and rectal temperature were recorded, and survival to 8 days was used to assess vitality. Increasing AA level reduced sow weight loss during lactation, but had no effect on vitality of the piglets or on sow health around farrowing. In the first 4 days after farrowing, fCHO and iCHO decreased feed intake, resulting in more back-fat loss. Farrowing process was not significantly affected by fiber type or content. PDS score worsened significantly with fCHO and iCHO. However, faecal consistency post-farrowing was improved with fCHO. Proportion of birth weight below 950 g increased with fCHO, iCHO being intermediate. However, neither piglet vitality nor growth pre-weaning responded to treatments. Altogether, the current results didn't support the need for increased AA, fCHO or iCHO in lactation diets.

Role of arcuate nucleus-kisspeptin/neurokinin b neurons in control of reproduction in cows

A.S.A. Hassaneen[1,2], M. Kato[2], Y. Suetomi[2], Y. Naniwa[2], T. Sasaki[2], N. Ieda[2], N. Inoue[2], K. Kimura[3], S. Oishi[4], N. Fujii[4], S. Matsuyama[5], R. Misu[4], S. Minabe[5], H. Tsukamura[2], F. Matsuda[2] and S. Ohkura[2]

[1]*Faculty of Veterinary Medicine, South Valley University, Theriogenology, Obstetrics and Artificial Insemination, Qena, Egypt,* [2]*Graduate School of Bioagricultural Sciences, Nagoya University, Laboratory of Animal Production Science, Furo-cho, Chikusa-ku, Nagoya, 464-8601, Nagoya, Japan,* [3]*Graduate School of Environmental and Life Science, Okayama University, Okayama University, 700-8530, Okayama, Japan,* [4]*Graduate School of Pharmaceutical Sciences, Kyoto University, 606-8501, Kyoto, Japan,* [5]*National Agriculture and Food Research Organization Institute of Livestock and Grassland Science, 329-2793, Nasushiobara, Japan; ahmed.hassaneen@vet.svu.edu.eg*

Many studies reported that kisspeptin neurons play an important role in control of gonadotropin-releasing hormone (GnRH) release in many species including cows. In mammals, including sheep, kisspeptin/neurokinin B (NKB) are expressed in the arcuate nucleus (ARC). It was found that, kisspeptin/NKB neurons play a role in the steroid feedback control of GnRH secretion. The aim of our study was to examine the role of kisspeptin/NKB neurons in control of reproduction in cows. In the first experiment, 8 heifers were used and these heifers were divided into 2 groups: follicular (n=4) and luteal (n=4) phase. The aim was to check whether kisspeptin/NKB neurons exist in the ARC of cows. Serial brain sections were double immunostained with antibodies against kisspeptin and NKB. In the second experiment, 17 Japanese Black beef cows were used. Our aim was to examine the effect of senktide, a neurokinin-3 receptor (NK3R) agonist on the luteinizing hormone (LH) release and ovarian function in cows. Cows were divided into follicular or luteal phase, and in each group cows were infused intravenously with senktide (30 or 300 nmol/min) or vehicle (n=4). Blood sampling were performed every 10 mins, and plasma samples were used to check the LH concentrations using radioimmunoassay. Ovarian ultrasonography was performed to examine the follicular growth and ovulation. Our study was the first to confirm that kisspeptin and NKB were co-expressed in the ARC but not in the preoptic area with higher expression in follicular phase than luteal phase. For the *in vivo* experiment, treatment with senktide 300 nmol/min resulted in a sustained increase in the plasma LH concentrations in both model. Early ovulation was detected in 2 out of 4 senktide 300 nmol/min treated cows in follicular phase but not in luteal phase. Taken together, we could conclude that kisspeptin/NKB neurons exist in the ARC of cows and that NKB/NK3R signaling is essential for GnRH release in cows.

The telemetric measurement of the reticulorumen and vaginal acidity and temperature of dairy cows

R. Antanaitis, G. Zamokas, A. Grigonis and V. Žilaitis

Lithuanian University of Health Sciences, Department of Non-Infectious Diseases, Tilžės str. 18, Kaunas, Lithuania, 47181, Lithuania; ramunas.antanaitis@lsmuni.lt

The objective of the research was to determine the relation of the reticulorumen and vaginal temperature and pH, and rectal temperature during the period after calving and assessing the potential risk of disease after calving (metritis, SARA). The pH and temperature of the contents of cows reticulorumens and uterus were measured using specific smaXtec boluses manufactured for animal care. The examination of the relation between the vaginal and rectal temperatures revealed a positive (r=0.352), statistically significant ($P<0.001$) correlation. A similar relation was found between the reticulorumen content temperature and the rectal temperature (r=0.257), ($P<0.0001$). A positive (r=0.253), statistically reliable ($P<0.0001$) correlation between the vaginal temperature and pH was found. A positive (r=0.277), statistically reliable ($P<0.0001$) correlation between the reticulorumen content pH and vaginal pH was found. A positive (r=0.385), statistically reliable ($P<0.0001$) correlation between the reticulorumen content temperature and vaginal temperature was found. In summary, it can be stated that the computerized measurement of reticulorumen temperature allows the evaluation of temperature changes in the rectum and the vagina. By measuring the reticulorumen pH, which may indicate changes of the vagina pH, which allows assessing the potential risk of disease after calving (metritis, SARA).

Proximal teat amputation in a Brown-Swiss cow with a severe udder oedema

P. Steckeler, C. Straub, M. Hipp and W. Petzl
Ludwig-Maximilians-University Munich, Clinic for Ruminants with Ambulance and Herd Health
Services, Sonnenstrasse 16, 85764 Oberschleissheim, Germany;
p.steckeler@med.vetmed.uni-muenchen.de

Teat injuries are common in dairy cows and occur most frequently around calving. During this period cows may show different grades of udder oedema. To avoid culling of the animal, immediate total amputation of the affected teat can often be the method with the best cost benefit. If the laceration of the teat affects the teat basis or distal parts of the udder, a proximal teat amputation is the recommended option. However this surgical method implies an increased risk of strong bleeding, since haemostasis with clamps is hindered. A 5 year old Brown-Swiss cow was presented at the Clinic for Ruminants, LMU Munich 2 days after calving. The right hind teat showed an open teat laceration, which had happened 8 h ago and besides complete destruction of distal parts of the teat also affected the teat base. Thus, a proximal teat amputation was required. The cow showed a severe udder oedema with a high grade firmness of the udder tissue. Prior to surgery, the cow was restrained and placed on her left side on an operation table, followed by treatment with 20 mg xylazine (i.v.), 3,000 mg enrofloxacine (i.v.) and 1,500 mg flunixine-meglumine (i.v.). The teat received local anaesthesia by circular infiltration in the region proximal of the injury with 40 ml of procaine 2%. Due to the severe udder oedema the general practice of positioning two Doyen's intestinal clamps proximal of the injury to reduce intraoperative bleeding and unwanted milk-flow was not possible. Therefore 6 temporary mass ligatures with silk (USP 6) were circularly applied in the udder tissue 3 cm around the teat base. The teat was removed with a scalpel in the region of the teat base and a cone shaped piece of tissue was removed to allow adaption of the outer skin. There were no complications with regards to intraoperative bleeding or milk flow. The cow received 300 mg cefquinome intracisternally. The glandular cistern was closed with a non-perforating horizontal mattress suture, the muscular tissue with a modified simple continuous suture (glyconate monofilament, absorbable, USP 3/0) and the skin with 6 U-shaped sutures (polyester, braided, non absorbable, USP 1). No postoperative bleeding could be observed after removing the 6 mass ligatures. Treatment with enrofloxacine and flunixine-meglumine was continued for the following 4 days. After 11 days the stiches in the outer skin were removed. The cow was released with a daily milk yield of 45 kg which was nearly 100% of her former milk production. Temporary mass ligatures can avoid intraoperative bleeding during proximal teat amputation. Thus in cases of severe udder oedema this surgical procedure can be performed and may avoid unwanted culling of cows.

Comparison of two different protocols for induction of parturition in heifers with or without estrad

H. Hamali, N. Mehrvar and A. Saberivand
The University of Tabriz, Clinical Sciences, 29 Bahman Boulivard, 5166616471 Tabriz, Iran;
hhamali@yahoo.com

Induction of parturition is one of the most important subjects in the dairy industry worldwide including Iran. Because of the use of imported semen from other countries, the need for induction of parturition is increasing. One of the most important side effects of induction of parturition is retained fetal membranes in cows. To study the effect of estradiol benzoate (Vetastrol, manufactured by Abureihan Company,Iran) on the rate of postpartum placental retention in heifers, a total number of 100 heifers from the dairy herds of Tabriz with similar nutrition and management systems were chosen and assigned into one of two groups. In the group A (Control, n=50) heifers that were a minimum of 270 days of pregnancy received 30 mg dexamethasone (Vetacoid, 50 ml vial, 1 ml containing: 2 mg dexamethasone sodium phosphate manufactured by Abureihan Company, Iran) intramuscularly. In the group B (Treatment, n=50) heifers received 30 mg dexamethasone plus 20 mg estradiol benzoate (Vetastrol, 10 ml vial, 1 ml containing 2 mg estradiol mono-benzoate manufactured by Abureihan Company, Iran) intramuscularly on the same days of pregnancy. The mean times for parturition were 41.5 h and 37.5 h in groups A and B respectively. 8 of 50 heifers in group A did not respond to induction of parturition and were omitted from the trial. 16 out of 42 heifers in group A had dystocia at the time of parturition (38%). All heifers in group B had successful parturition and only 9 heifers showed difficulty in calving. 33 heifers (78%) from group A and 32 heifers (64%) from the group B showed retention of fetal membranes after parturition. The differences between two groups were statistically significant ($P \leq 0.05$). In conclusion, our results indicated that induction of parturition by estradiol benzoate and dexamethasone together is superior to dexamethasone alone because of the less retention of fetal membranes, easy calving and shorter time from induction to parturition.

The effects of FSH treatment in Ovsynch protocol on pregnancy rate in dairy cows

G. Yilmazbas-Mecitoglu[1], A. Gumen[1], A. Keskin[1], E. Karakaya[1], U. Tasdemir[2] and A. Alkan[1]
[1]Uludag University Faculty of Veterinary Medicine, Obstetrics and Gynecology, Animal Hospital Gorukle Campus, 16059 Bursa, Turkey; [2]Aksaray University, Vocational School of Technical Sciences, 68100 Aksaray, Turkey; gulnazy@gmail.com

The aim of the study was to determine the effects of FSH treatment at specific times after first GnRH administration of the ovsynch protocol on pregnancy rate to timed AI (TAI). Primiparous and multiparous Holstein-Fresian (n=345) and Swedish Red (n=38) cows were used. Cows were randomly assigned to one of four experimental groups. Control group (n=212) recieved ovsynch protocol; the first GnRH (Buserelin acetate, 10 mcg) of ovsynch and seven days after GnRH, PGF2α (Cloprostenol, 500 mcg) was administered. A second GnRH treatment was administered 56 h after PGF2α and all cows were inseminated at a fixed time 16-18 h after the final GnRH treatment using frozen thawed semen. Group FSH3 (n=92), FSH4 (n=88) and FSH3-4 (n=91) received same TAI protocol with the addition of FSH (follicle stimulating hormone, 35 İE) at day 3, 4 or both day 3 and 4 after the first GnRH administration, respectively. Ultrasonographic examinations were done at the beginning of the study to determine the cyclicity of the cows, seven days later GnRH to determine ovulatory response on the ovary, at the time of TAI to determine follicle number and to measure ovulatory follicle diameter, 7 days after TAI to determine of ovulation of the dominant follicle (ovulatory response to second GnRH), at 31 and 62 days after TAI to determine pregnancy rates (PR) and accessory CL. DIM, BCS, milk production, ovulation number, ovulation responses to first and second GnRH, accessory CL at 31 and 62 days, PR on 31 and 62 days did not differ among groups. However follicle number ($P=0.03$) and follicle diameter ($P=0.02$) were different among groups. In conclusion, FSH administration was not found beneficial after first GnRH administration of Ovsynch protocol to improve PR and reduce embryonic loss.

Study on the effect of retained fetal membranes on the reproductive performance in dairy cattle

I. Elbawab[1], M. Elbehiry[2], M. Marey[2], K. Metwally[1] and F. Hussein[1]
[1] Faculty of Veterinary Medicine, Alexandria University, Theriogenology, Alexandria, Egypt, 22758, Egypt, [2] Faculty of Veterinary Medicine, Damanhour University, Theriogenology, Damanhour-Elbehira, 22511, Egypt; behairy_2010@yahoo.com

Postpartum disorders such as retained fetal membranes (RFM) adversely affect reproductive performance in dairy cows. This study aimed to investigate the effect of RFM on the reproductive performance in dairy cattle. A total of 43 multiparous Holstein dairy cows were used in this study. Cows were closely observed after parturition for descent of the fetal membranes then assigned into one of 3 groups, group I (n=26) as a control group with normal expulsion of fetal membranes ($\leq$12 h postpartum), group II (n=8) suffered from RFM with manual removal and group III (n=9) with RFM left without any intervention. Fetal membranes were expelled after 4.92$\pm$0.59 h, 26.12$\pm$8.56 h, and 44.55$\pm$5.70 h postpartum in group I, II, and III, respectively. The color, odor and duration of lochia discharge were recorded for all cows from parturition until complete cessation. All cows were examined rectally for uterine involution and ovarian resumption of cyclicity from calving to first service. Estrus signs were observed twice daily by a well-experienced herdsman. Cows in estrus were artificially inseminated up to 3 inseminations until conception. Our results showed that RFM significantly ($P<0.01$) prolonged the mean duration of lochia discharge compared with normal cows (group I, II, and III were 10.5$\pm$0.60, 19.62$\pm$1.77 and 15.88$\pm$1.22 days respectively). Moreover, RFM changed the odor and color of Lochia discharge from odorless and glassy from the 7th day postpartum in normal cows into grayish brown or grayish white with offensive odor in cows with RFM. Involution of the gravid and non-gravid horns was significantly delayed ($P<0.01$) in RFM cows with or without manual removal when compared with normal cows. Restoration of ovarian follicular activity occurred after 16.73$\pm$0.57, 22.00$\pm$1.74 and 18.88$\pm$1.35 days for group I, II, and III, respectively. Respective values for the first observed estrus (standing estrus) in the three groups were 50.61$\pm$3.79, 59.50$\pm$2.68 and 51.00$\pm$4.15 days. The average open days was 68.54$\pm$4.17, 129.13$\pm$13.04 and 116.33$\pm$12.27 days for normal cows, retained placenta with and without manual removal respectively with highly significant difference ($P<0.0001$) between the three groups. In conclusion, retained fetal membranes associated with uterine infection adversely affected uterine involution, ovarian activity and days open and decreased the reproductive performance of dairy cows. Manual removal of RFM increased this adverse effect.

Optimising welfare and economic performance in alternative farrowing and lactation systems

E.M. Baxter[1] and S.A. Edwards[2]
[1]SRUC, Animal Behavior and Welfare, Animal and Veterinary Sciences Group, West Mains Road, Edinburgh, EH9 3JG, United Kingdom, [2]Newcastle University, School of Agriculture, Food and Rural Development, Agriculture Building, Newcastle Upon Tyne, NE1 7RU, United Kingdom; emma.baxter@sruc.ac.uk

Within the pig industry one of the major issues involving trade-offs between welfare and production goals involves housing of pregnant and farrowing sows. Confinement of the sow during pregnancy (sow stalls) and lactation (farrowing crates) are good examples of where a mismatch between biological needs and building design results in a welfare compromise which is a continuing focus for public concern. The EU-wide partial ban on sow gestation stalls came into force in 2013. Presently there is no similar overall ban of farrowing crates, though there is growing societal pressure to abolish individual confinement systems. Producers are often reluctant to voluntarily change, with many citing valid concerns about loss in performance, increased capital, running and labour costs and issues with operator safety. Thus the design challenge is to construct a suitable alternative system that reconciles a 'triangle of needs' belonging to the farmer, the sow and her piglets. Difficulties arise because of various conflicts between these three parties (e.g. sow vs farmer: space needed for nest-building vs space needed to maximise herd size) and within these three parties (e.g. sow: maximising the survival of her current litter vs maintaining condition for future litters). Resolving these conflicts and designing a system that maximises sow and piglet welfare whilst maintaining an economically efficient and sustainable business is the target. Research efforts have led to successful development of loose farrowing systems delivering high performance and high welfare. Key to success has been recognising that allowing the display of species-typical behaviours contributes to the biological fitness of the animal. Biological fitness encompasses important economic performance indicators including; reproductive potential, number and quality of offspring produced and ability to rear offspring. Once physiological and behavioural needs of animals which are sensitive to the physical environment (e.g. nest-building in peri-parturient sows) have been identified they need to be translated into design criteria (e.g. dimensions of physical space) for builders of livestock housing. The details of these criteria are crucial to success. Finally in order to encourage uptake and sustainability of high welfare systems it is critical to achieve consistent performance. Therefore system optimisation should be accompanied by optimisation of both human inputs (i.e. through augmentation of management) and animal inputs (i.e. through genetic selection strategies).

Environmental and social enrichment reduces susceptibility to co-infection in pigs

I.D.E. Van Dixhoorn[1], I. Reimert[2], J.E. Bolhuis[2], P.W.G. Groot Koerkamp[1], B. Kemp[2] and N. Stockhofe-Zurwieden[3]
[1]Wageningen UR, Livestock Research, De Elst 1, 6708 WD Wageningen, the Netherlands, [2]Wageningen UR, Adaptation Physiology Group, De Elst 1, 6708 WD Wageningen, the Netherlands, [3]Wageningen UR, Central Veterinary Institute, Edelhertweg 15, 8219 PH Lelystad, the Netherlands; ingrid.vandixhoorn@wur.nl

A combination of viral and bacterial pathogens and environmental factors, can cause porcine respiratory disease complex (PRDC) in pigs. PRDC leads to diminished growth, health problems or death as well as to economic losses. Anti-microbial drugs are often used against bacterial infections. However, resistance against antibiotics is of growing concern. As stress can result in impaired immune protection, psycho-neuroimmunological intervention may prove to be a successful approach to diminish the susceptibility to diseases. Modern pig production is characterized by high stock density and stimulus poor housing conditions. The effects of rearing under barren conditions on behaviour, fear and stress are well known. However, little information is available on the influence of positive conditions on susceptibility to infectious disease. This study was designed to investigate the effect of environmental and social enrichment on disease susceptibility in pigs using a co-infection model of porcine reproductive and respiratory virus (PRRSV) and *Actinobacillus pleuropneumoniae*. These two pathogens are frequently involved in PRDC. Four groups of 7 piglets grew up under barren conditions and four groups of 7 piglets were raised under enriched conditions. In the enriched groups a combination of established social and environmental enrichment factors were introduced, that have proven to enhance welfare. At the age of 44 days, two groups of the barren (BH) and two groups of the enriched housed (EH) pigs were infected with PRRSV followed 8 days later by *A. pleuropneumoniae*. The other two groups served as control groups. We tested if differences in susceptibility in terms of pathological and clinical outcome were related to the different housing conditions, and if this was reflected in differences in behavioural, immunological and physiological states in the pigs. EH pigs showed a faster clearance of viral PRRSV RNA in serum ($P<0.05$) and had histologically 2.8 fold less typical PRRSV related scores in the lungs ($P<0.05$). The total number of EH pigs with lesions in the lungs post mortally was 8 fold ($P<0.05$) lower and the lesions showed a lower total pathologic tissue damage score (2.1 fold, $P<0.05$) than BH pigs. Moreover, the EH pigs showed less stress related behaviour and differed immunologically and physiologically from BH pigs. We conclude that a combination of environmental and social enrichment reduces disease susceptibility to co-infection of PRRSV and *A. pleuropneumoniae*.

Cost-efficiency of animal welfare in broiler prodcution systems

E. Gocsik[1], S.D. Brooshooft[1], I.C. De Jong[2] and H.W. Saatkamp[1]
[1]Wageningen University, Business Economics Group, Hollandseweg 1, 6706 KN Wageningen, the Netherlands, [2]Wageningen University Livestock Research, Elst 1, 6708 WD, Wageningen, the Netherlands; eva.gocsik@wur.nl

Broiler producers operate in a highly competitive and cost-price driven environment. In addition, in recent years the societal pressure to improve animal welfare (AW) in broiler production systems is increasing. Hence, from an economic and decision making point of view, the cost-efficiency of improvement in AW obtained from a certain production system is of great importance. Therefore, the aim of this paper was to analyze the contribution of four different production systems to overall AW and the cost-efficiency of increased AW at the farm level. Cost-efficiency was calculated as the ratio of the change in the level of animal welfare and the change in the level of production costs compared to the level of conventional system (i.e. legal minimum standards). The level of AW was measured by the Welfare Quality index score (WQ index score) calculated on the basis of data collected in 168 flocks in the Netherlands, United Kingdom and Italy within the Welfare Quality® project. On the basis of systems attributes, three main segments of production systems are distinguished, i.e. conventional, middle-market and top-market systems. The middle-market and top-market systems use a slow growing breed. Stocking density ranges from 25 to 31 kg/m2 in middle-market systems and from 21 to 27.5 kg/m2 in top-market systems. In the middle-market systems, a covered veranda is provided to the chickens, whereas in the top-market systems chickens have access to an outdoor range. Total production costs were calculated for each production system using a deterministic economic model. Results show that the middle-market systems, such as the Dutch Volwaard and Puur & Eerlijk systems, had the highest WQ index score (736), whereas the conventional system had the lowest (577). Moreover, the WQ index score of extensive outdoor (733) and organic systems (698) was below that of the middle-market systems. Three system attributes contributed most to AW in all systems, i.e. broiler type, stocking density and length of the dark period. With respect to production costs, broiler chickens kept in conventional system were produced at the lowest costs, followed by the middle-market, the extensive outdoor, and the organic systems. With regard to cost-efficiency, when shifting from conventional to an alternative system, middle-market systems (i.e. Volwaard and Puur & Eerlijk; 8.37) outperformed the extensive outdoor (3.90) and organic systems (1.03). Overall, it can be concluded that the middle-market systems could be attractive for farmers due to their high cost-efficiency, a higher WQ index score and the flexibility to revert to the conventional system.

Selection for or against feather pecking: what are the consequences?

J.A.J. Van Der Eijk[1,2], A. Lammers[2], B. Kemp[2], M. Naguib[1] and T.B. Rodenburg[1]
[1]Wageningen University, Behavioural Ecology, De Elst 1, 6708 WD Wageningen, the Netherlands,
[2]Wageningen University, Adaptation Physiology, De Elst 1, 6708 WD Wageningen, the Netherlands;
jerine.vandereijk@wur.nl

Feather pecking is a major welfare and economic concern for the worldwide egg production industry. This behaviour involves hens pecking and pulling at feathers or tissue of conspecifics, causing feather and tissue damage and it can even lead to mortality of victims. Beak trimming is currently used to limit damage and mortality from feather pecking. However, with the expected ban on beak trimming in many EU countries, it is crucial to find alternative solutions to control this damaging behaviour. Certain behavioural traits, such as fearfulness, have been related to the occurrence of feather pecking. However, it is unknown whether selection for or against feather pecking affects behaviour and development in young hens. The aim of this study was to evaluate the effects of selection for and against feather pecking on feather pecking, fearfulness and growth. We used genetic lines selected for high (HFP) and low (LFP) feather pecking and an unselected control (CON) line to identify effects of selection on behaviour and growth characteristics. Lines were housed separately in groups of 19 hens per pen, with 8 pens per line. Group size was reduced by 2-3 hens at 0, 5 and 10 weeks of age. Hens were weighed at 0, 4, 9 and 14 weeks of age, and tested in a tonic immobility (TI) test at 13 weeks of age. Feather pecking observations were performed at 8 and 9 weeks of age for 30 min per pen. Data were analysed using mixed or generalized mixed models with fixed effect of line and random effect of pen nested within batch. As expected, more hens from the HFP line were classified as feather peckers compared to CON and LFP lines (HFP=19.82%, CON=6.80% and LFP=4.95%, $F_{2,290}=3.59$, $P=0.0288$). The HFP line had a shorter TI duration compared to CON and LFP lines (HFP=84.39 s, CON=142.78 s and LFP=140.31 s, $F_{2,189}=6.09$, $P=0.0027$). Interestingly, LFP hens had lower body weight compared to HFP and CON hens at 0 ($F_{2,432}=8.27$, $P=0.0003$), 4 ($F_{2,359}=6.26$, $P=0.0021$), 9 ($F_{2,290}=10.51$, $P<0.0001$) and 14 weeks of age ($F_{2,223}=14.86$, $P<0.0001$). Furthermore, the LFP line had a lower growth rate compared to CON and HFP lines between 0 and 14 weeks of age ($F_{2,225}=14.12$, $P<0.0001$). Thus, HFP hens were less fearful compared to CON and LFP hens. Furthermore, selection against feather pecking seems to have a negative effect on body weight and growth rate at young ages. In conclusion, our results suggest that selection for or against feather pecking not only affects feather pecking, but also other behavioural characteristics and development in young hens. These results help to better understand possible consequences of genetic selection for reduced feather pecking.

Keeping pigs with intact tails: from science to practice

M. Kluivers-Poodt, N. Dirx, C.M.C. Van Der Peet, A. Hoofs, W.W. Ursinus, J.E. Bolhuis and G.F.V. Van Der Peet
Wageningen University and Research Centre, De Elst 1, 6708WD Wageningen, the Netherlands; marion.kluivers@wur.nl

Despite EU legislation, in intensive pig farming most pigs are tail docked. Several Dutch business and NGO parties have designed the Declaration of Dalfsen, a road map towards intact tails. First step is a demonstration keeping pigs with intact tails in a conventional system, aimed at closing the gap between science and practice and relieving the anxiety and scepticism among pig farmers. In 2014 and 2015, 117 litters with 1,428 animals were not tail docked. Farm risk factors related to (tail) biting were assessed and optimized. Environmental enrichment was provided, using a variety of materials: several kinds of roughage, rope, wood, burlap sacks. Caretakers were trained to recognize early signs of biting behaviour and to implement curative measures. Tails were inspected and scored in detail at 3, 4 and 9 weeks of age and before slaughter. Pigs were inspected twice daily for tail posture and tail wounds. In case of a wound, a check list was filled out and curative measures implemented. At 3 weeks of age, 39% had bite marks and 9% a tail wound, at 4 weeks this was 38 and 15%, at 9 weeks 16 and 14%, before slaughter 5 and 12%. During the growing and finishing phase curative measures had to be provided at some point to 10% of the animals and in 22 resp. 44% of the pens. In case of an obsessive biter, numbers of bitten pigs in the pen were high. A quick identification and removal of the biter proved essential and effective. In the course of the project, caretakers developed a higher level of alertness regarding (early) signs of biting, and a more active approach towards required measures. However, tail biting appeared throughout the entire course of the project. To enhance proper care during shifts of caretakers, a traffic light system was implemented to indicate litters at risk. Labour required for adequate monitoring and providing materials was higher than expected and the use of some enrichment materials encountered practical problems. The key in keeping pigs with intact tails is not looking more, but looking differently at the pigs. Training and coaching animal keepers is the starting point. Biting behaviour was already present in the farrowing pen, stressing the importance of 'starting early' with preventive measures. Early signs of biting were not always recognized or may not always be present. Therefore, effective curative measures are essential when keeping pigs with intact tails. Hospital pens proved mandatory to separate biters or victims. All present and gained (international) knowledge regarding keeping pigs with intact tails needs to be incorporated in an educational programme for pig farmers and farm advisors, to enable a responsible transition towards intact tails.

Genetic association between early calfhood health status and subsequent performance of dairy cows

M. Mahmoud, T. Yin and S. König

University of Kassel, Animal breeding, Nordbahnhof st. 1a, 37213 Witzenhausen, Germany; m.mahmoud@uni-kassel.de

Information from 31,359 of Holstein dairy cows was collected from 43 herds in Germany in the five years from 2010 to 2015, to estimate heritabilities, phonotypic correlation and genetic correlations among calfhood health status and functional and production traits for the same animal at first-lactation period (as a cow). The selected calfhood health traits were calf general health status, calf respiratory disease, and calf scours; The selected first-lactation functional traits were cow general health status, cow respiratory disease, cow scours, cow fertility, cow lameness, cow mastitis and cow metabolic disorder; First-lactation production traits were milk yield at the first test-day, milk yield at the second test-day, fat percentage at the first test-day, fat percentage at the second test-day, protein percentage at the first test-day, protein percentage at the second test-day, fat yield at the first test-day, fat yield at the second test-day, protein yield at the first test-day, protein yield at the second test-day, average milk yield in first lactation period, fat to protein ratio at the first test-day, fat to protein ratio at the second test-day. Random regression models are used in the analysis. Four generations have been traced back from the current population, and the variance components were estimated using a pedigree of 94,168 animals. The results show low heritabilities (0.06 and 0.07) for calf health traits and low heritability (0.05 to 0.12) for first-lactation functional traits and relatively moderate heritability (0.12 to 0.33) for first-lactation production traits. The genetic relationship between calfhood health traits and first-lactation functional traits suggest that, healthy and well-functioning cows are the result of hygienic selected young calves with good management before they entering the milking herd. Despite the known antagonistic genetic relationship between calfhood health traits and first-lactation production performance, not all detailed aspects of productive performance exhibited an unfavorable relationship. Thus if selection for improving some production traits were practiced, weighting all traits by their appropriate health-economic values would be required.

Enrichment materials for intensively-farmed pigs: from review to preview
M.B.M. Bracke
Wageningen UR, Livestock Research, De Elst 1, 6708 WD Wageningen, the Netherlands;
marc.bracke@wur.nl

Tail biting is a well-known production disease in intensively-farmed pigs raising concern for animal welfare, e.g. related to the practice of routine tail docking. To reduce tail biting pigs are provided with enrichment materials. EU legislation requires that pigs have permanent access to a sufficient quantity of material to enable proper investigation and manipulation activities. In order to meet this directive many pigs are provided with a metal chain with or without a rather indestructible object attached to the chain. The European commission is planning to revise current guidelines as to what constitutes adequate enrichment, apparently moving into the direction of the status-quo in welfare schemes. Building on extensive previous work at Wageningen UR Livestock Research, especially on the modelling of pig enrichment (the so-called RICHPIG model) a review is presented of our current state of knowledge. In addition, an outline is given as to how so-called AMI-sensors, measuring Animal-Material Interactions (AMI) (semi-)automatically, can be used to assess the pig's need for enrichment, also in relation to aspects associated with health status, such as feed restriction, biting wounds and streptococcus infection. It is suggested that the use of chains with or without rather indestructible materials such as pipes, balls or (hard)wood is generally inadequate to enrich the pens of intensively-farmed pigs. An evolutionary mechanism appears to be underlying the causation of multifactorial welfare problems in general, the issues of enrichment, tail biting and tail docking in pigs in particular. In this respect ongoing selection for increased resource efficiency has been exerting a profound impact on livestock production. Various routes are explored as to how persistent welfare problems may be resolved, including a method that has been called Intelligent Natural Design (IND).

A survey of straw use and tail biting in Swedish undocked pig farms

T. Wallgren, R. Westin and S. Gunnarsson
Swedish University of Agricultural Sciences, Dept. of Animal Environment and Health, Inst för
husdjurens miljö och hälsa, Box 234, 53223 Skara, Sweden; torun.wallgren@slu.se

Tail biting is a common problem in todays' pig production, affecting production and welfare. As tail biting behaviour is more prominent in systems with no or limited access manipulable material, it has been considered related to exploratory behaviours. Tail docking, commonly used as tail biting prevention, is a painful procedure that can decrease pig welfare does not eliminate the tail biting behaviour. Although tail docking is not accepted as a routine procedure according to the EU Directive 2008/120/EC it is still a common practise within the EU, which is why other measures to reduce tail biting behaviour are needed. In Sweden, tail docking is banned and tail biting must be reduced otherwise. Furthermore, Swedish legislation banned fully slatted floors and demands pigs to have access to manipulable material. In order to investigate the prevalence of tail biting in Sweden and the relationship with provision of straw, we performed a telephone survey in nursery (n=46) and finishing pig (n=43) farms. Farmers were interviewed regarding straw usage (e.g. daily ratios) and tail biting (e.g. frequency). All participating farmers gave access to manipulable material and 98% used straw. The median straw ration reported by farmers was 29 g/pig/day (min: 8 g, max: 85 g) in nursery and 50 g/pig/day (9 g, 225 g) in finishing farms when excluding deep litter systems. Farmers reported having observed tail bitten pigs, at any time, in 50% of nursery and 88% of finishing pig farms. Of these, tail bitten pigs were reported to be found ≤2 times/year (78%), 3-6 times/year(17%) or monthly (4%) in nursery and ≤2 times/year (21%), 3-6 times/year (37%), monthly (34%) or weekly (8%) in finishing farms. Finishing farmers reported on average 1.6% tail bitten pigs/batch (0.1-6.5%), which is in line with abattoir data. Spearman rank correlation was used for statistical analysis. Increased straw ration was correlated with decreased reported tail biting frequency in finishing farms (r=-0.39, P=0.03, n=31), and a tendency for this was found in nursery farms (r=-0.33, P=0.08, n=29) when deep litter systems were included. In finishing farms, excluding deep litter systems, an increased tail biting frequency observed by farmers was correlated to the percentage of tail bitten pigs (r=0.64, P≤0.001, n=33), indicating that an increased frequency of tail biting reported may be associated with more pens affected at outbreaks. Even though provided straw rations were quite small (i.e. 30-50 g/pig/day), this amount of straw may provide pigs with enough occupation to limit tail biting outbreaks. We conclude that tail biting can be kept at a low level (ca 2%) in partly slatted flooring systems, without tail docking, by suppluing straw.

Prevalence of production diseases in organic dairy herds in Germany, Spain, France, and Sweden

M. Krieger[1], A. Madouasse[2,3], K. Sjöström[4], U. Emanuelson[4], I. Blanco-Penedo[5], J.E. Duval[2,3], N. Bareille[2,3], C. Fourichon[2,3] and A. Sundrum[1]
[1]University of Kassel, 37213, Witzenhausen, Germany, [2]INRA, 44307, Nantes, France, [3]LUNAM Université, Oniris, 44307, Nantes, France, [4]SLU, 75007, Uppsala, Sweden, [5]IRTA, 17121, Monells, Spain; margret.krieger@uni-kassel.de

Organic farming in Europe is governed by Regulation (EC) 834/2007 and standards of private label organisations. Whereas compliance with the production rules is inspected on a regular basis, there is no monitoring of the fulfilment of the organic principles, particularly the principle of health. The purpose of this study was to assess the level of production diseases in organic dairy herds across Europe. National milk records and animal movement data were retrieved and a selection of the lactating cows was scored for lameness according to the Welfare Quality® protocol on a sample of farms. Prevalence of production diseases were calculated using sets of herd-level indicators and common R scripts. In total, 192 farms participated, i.e. 60 in Germany, 23 in Spain, 54 in France, and 55 in Sweden. Herd size expressed as cow-years ranged from 7 to 377; smallest in Spain (median [m]=30) and largest in Sweden (m=68). In all countries Holstein was the predominant breed with shares of 100% in Spain, 53% in France, and 41% in Germany as well as Sweden. Median energy-corrected milk yield was 6,588 kg in Germany, 5,742 kg in Spain, 6,378 kg in France, and 8,979 kg in Sweden. Herd prevalence of subclinical mastitis, defined as composite milk samples above a somatic cell count of 100,000 cells/ml, had a range of 19-94%; lowest in Sweden (m=44%) and highest in Spain (m=58%). Across countries a median of 10% of animals were at risk of ketosis, diagnosed by a fat-to-protein ratio >1.5 during the first 100 days of lactation (range 0 – 45%). Milk fat percentage <3.0 after 30 days in milk was used as indicator for subacute ruminal acidosis (SARA). Herd prevalence ranged from 0 to 42% with an overall median of 3% and Spain deviating the most (m=15%). Prevalence of prolonged calving interval (>400 days) was highest in Spain (m=63%) and lowest in Germany (m=36%) with a range of 4-91%. Overall (moderate and severe) lameness prevalence ranged from 0 to 79% and was lowest in Sweden (m=4%) and highest in France (m=23%). It can be concluded that the level of production diseases varies widely between organic dairy farms in Europe with a considerable proportion of farms not meeting the aim of good animal health. The results call for new, improved strategies to achieve good animal health in organic dairy systems, starting with unified monitoring procedures. This project has received funding from the EU FP7 for research, technological development and demonstration under grant agreement n° 311824 (IMPRO).

Effect of hatching conditions on indicators of welfare and health in broiler chickens

I.C. De Jong[1], H. Gunnink[1], P. De Gouw[2], F. Leijten[2], M. Raaijmakers[1,3], L. Zoet[1,3], E. Wolfs[2], L.F.J. Van De Ven[2] and H. Van Den Brand[3]
[1]*Wageningen UR Livestock Research, Animal Welfare, P.O. Box 338, 6700 AH Wageningen, the Netherlands,* [2]*Vencomatic Group, P.O. Box 160, 5520 AD Eersel, the Netherlands,* [3]*Wageningen University, Adaptation Physiology, P.O. Box 338, 6700 AH Wageningen, the Netherlands; ingrid.dejong@wur.nl*

On-farm hatching of broiler chickens is increasingly applied, because farmers report improved performance compared to broilers hatched at the hatchery. However, there is little scientific evidence for these effects. Aim of the study was to find evidence for long-lasting effects of hatching conditions on performance and welfare of broiler chickens. Broilers hatched at the hatchery (n=16 control flocks) or on-farm (X-treck system, n=16 flocks). Each X-treck flock was paired to a control flock from similar parent stock, reared in identical houses and subjected to similar management. In the X-treck, eggs are transferred to the stable at d18 of incubation and hatch in the stable. Chicks have immediate access to feed and water. Chicks from the hatchery received their first feed and water when they arrived at the farm. Indicators of welfare were measured at d0 (arrival of hatchery chicks), d21 and just before slaughter. Analysis of variance was used to test effects of treatment and age; data were transformed if necessary. X-treck broilers were heavier at d0 compared to control broilers ($P<0.01$) due to immediate access to feed and water after hatching. Quality of X-treck chicks was impaired compared to control chicks, as indicated by on average a worse navel and leg quality ($P=0.01$), which might be due to selection of chicks at the hatchery, which did not happen in the X-treck system. Control chicks showed a more stressful response (more vocalisations) in a novel environment test at d0 compared to X-treck chicks ($P<0.01$), but there were no treatment differences at d21. No treatment differences in gait score at d21 and at slaughter age were found, indicating that hatching conditions did not affect lameness. X-treck broilers had less foot pad dermatitis at d21 and slaughter age ($P<0.05$) and had numerically better hock burn scores at slaughter age than control broilers ($P=0.56$). X-treck broilers were more dirty at d21 and at slaughter age than control broilers ($P=0.08$). Litter quality was better in X-treck houses than in control houses, which seems to be in contradiction to bird cleanliness but in agreement with foot and hock scores. Farm records of the majority of flocks indicated a lower rejection rate at slaughter and a lower mortality for X-treck flocks compared to control flocks, although these figures need to be confirmed in the final analysis. Thus, first results of this study indicate that effects of hatching conditions on welfare of broiler chickens may indeed be long-lasting.

Bovine practitioner survey: can a new obstetrical instrument really make the difference?

F. Schlederer[1] and A. Wehrend[2]
[1]Private Practice, Lichtegg 1, 4770 Andorf, Austria, [2]Institute for Veterinary Gynecology and Obstetrics, Frankfurter Strasse 106, 35392 Giessen, Germany; vet.lichtegg@speed.at

Dystocia in cattle affects up to 50% of primiparous and 30% of adult cows1. Obstetrics are crucial in order to reduce stillbirth rates. GYNstick2,3,4, a new tool for treating dystocia, has been available for practitioners for almost 3 years. A survey was conducted among 49 German and 5 Austrian practitioners to obtain feedback about their experience with this instrument and their recommendations for its use. Veterinarians were chosen based on their practical experience with this new instrument for at least 1 year. The data analysis compared the veterinarians experiences by gender, age and frequency of dystocia interventions. The majority (n=30, 56.6%) of the respondents were female vets. Most of the practitioners (64%) stated that GYNstick was recommended to them by another colleague. Twenty-six percent were informed by advertising and 20% by scientific literature. Females recommended the tool more often than males (70 vs 57%, $P=0.23$; χ^2 test). For 83% of the responders, the correction of a twisted uterus was the most frequent indication for using the instrument. Correction of mal-positionings was the second most frequent indication (65%). Females used the GYNstick more frequently for malpositioned calves than males ($P=0.04$, χ^2). The third most common indication was displaced extremities (69%)´, the fouth one (95%) the avoidance of fetotomy. Most veterinarians (92.5%) think that the instrument reduces the duration of dystocia, without differences between males and females ($P=0.9$, χ^2). Forty-three percent of the vets estimated a 30% time reduction. Forty-four percent estimated a 30-50% time reduction. Approximately 2/3 (65%) of the vets felt that the instrument did not impact the number of live calves born. For the remaining veterinarians, 24% thought that number of calves born alive was 30% greater after implementing this tool. Nine percent of veterinarians estimated an increase in live calves of 50% (no gender differences; $P=0.1$, χ^2). 84% of the practitioners are convinced that the instrument is a more effective life-saver than traditional obstetrical instruments. 45% of the practitioners replied that up to 30% and more stillborns can be avoided by using the tool. 'Making life easier' is a very important aspect for practitioners. All users are convinced that it is less exhausting in comparison to other tools or manual interventions. In addition, 21% said that muscle efforts are reduced by 50-80%. Interestingly, this outcome was not impacted by sex of the veterinarian ($P=0.1$, χ^2). All respondents replied that they would recommend (81% full agreement, 19%, recommend if asked) the tool to their colleagues.

Dairy cow metabolic status management through productivity and biochemical compounds of milk

I. Sematovica and L. Liepa
Latvia University of Agriculture, Faculty of Veterinary Medicine, Helmana 8, Jelgava, 3004, Latvia; isem@inbox.lv

In large production farms, it is sometimes difficult to detect the management mistakes and economical losses associated with management problems. The aim of our study was to analyse the milk productivity results among healthy cows and cows predisposed to metabolic diseases (subacute rumen acidosis (SARA), ketosis) in a management group. The study was conducted as a part of the government-funded project VP29. Interconnections between the milk yield and milk biochemical indices (fat, protein, lactose and urea) were analysed in a 600 dairy cows' herd with a milk yield 7,500 kg per cow and affected by SARA and ketosis. Data were acquired in a 12 month period from cows in the group with an increasing production curve (from day 4 to day 60 in lactation). Cows were fed with a total mixed ration in this group, the mean number of cows stayed at 93±7 while the number of places at the feed table was 70. The monthly milk samples were tested biochemically in an accredited milk testing laboratory. The test results from 1,118 cows were divided in three groups: Group 1 (G1): cows predisposed to SARA with fat/protein ratio (F/P) <0.9 (61 cows, from which 95.6% had milk fat below 3%); Group 2 (G2): healthy cows with optimum F/P 1.2-1.6; and Group 3 (G3): cows predisposed to ketosis with F/P>1.6 (54 cows, from which 76% had milk fat above 5%). The amount of energy-corrected milk (ECM) was calculated using the formula: ECM = milk kg × [(0.383 × fat %) + (0.242 × protein %) + 0.7832] / 3.140. Data was statistically analysed with computer programs MS Excel and SPSS. The productivity of cows within the group with an increasing production curve was highly variable: from 23.6 to 65.6 kg per day and F/P ratio was in range from 0.39 to 2.58. In G1, the fat content in milk was 2.5±0.33% and, the milk yield per day was significantly ($P<0.01$) higher in G1 than in G2 and G3: 45.5±7.5 kg, 41.3±8.44 kg and 38.4±11.9 kg respectively. Whereas, in G1, ECM 36.23±6.17 kg was significantly ($P<0.001$) lower, but milk urea concentration 32.66±9.18 mg/dl had tendency to be higher than in G2, 41.5±8.64 kg and 30.3±7.00 mg/dl respectively, and in G3, 43.4±12.8 kg and 30.3±7.0 mg/dl respectively. We detected significant average positive correlation (r=0.72; $P<0.01$) between F/P and the difference between milk productivity kg and ECM. The grouping of cows in free stall facilities in excessively crowded groups based solely on physiological period of lactation is not acceptable. Thus the cows are predisposed to metabolic disorders, like SARA and ketosis, and economic losses occur from ineffective use of feed protein resources. SARA predisposed cows are producing less ECM than milk productivity kg, but ketosis predisposed conversely.

Shoulder ulcers in sows; systemic response and the effect of ketoprofen medication

M. Nystén[1], T. Orro[2] and O. Peltoniemi[1]
[1]Faculty of Veterinary Medicine, University of Helsinki, Production Animal Medicine, Leissantie 43, 04920 Saarentaus, Finland, [2]Institute of Veterinary Medicine and Animal Sciences, Estonian University of Life Sciences, Clinical Veterinary Medicine, Kreutzwaldi 62, 51014 Tartu, Estonia; maria.polso@helsinki.fi

Several predisposing factors and aspects of the pathogenesis of shoulder ulcers in lactating sows are known, but many other aspects still require further study. The aim of our study was to assess the systemic response to shoulder ulcers, and the effect of pain relief with non-steroidal anti-inflammatory medication (ketoprofen) on the incidence of shoulder ulcers in a Finnish porcine farm. Our study hypothesis was that relief of the pain associated with farrowing and the early lactation, by means of NSAID medication, would have a preventive effect on the formation of shoulder ulcers. In the double-blinded study, 144 sows received either ketoprofen (3 mg/kg, n=71) or placebo (n=73) as intramuscular injection for two days after parturition. Sows were clinically examined before farrowing and after weaning. The examination included back and shoulder fat measurement, body condition scoring and grading of shoulder ulcer (grades 0-4). In addition, the sows were assessed weekly for the presence of shoulder ulcer. Haptoglobin and albumin were measured from serum samples taken 12 days (mean 11, variation 4-14) after farrowing (n=37). Haptoglobin was analyzed with the hemoglobin-binding method and albumin with the colorimetric method. Study results were analyzed with linear regression model for associations between haptoglobin, albumin and shoulder ulcers, where a three levels ordered response variable for shoulder ulcers was used (no ulcers, unilateral ulcers and bilateral ulcers). For risk factors and the effect of ketoprofen treatment, a random ordered logistic model was used. There was a significant decrease in albumin level and increase in haptoglobin level in sows with bilater shoulder ulcers (n=6) when compared to sows with no shoulder ulcer (n=22, $P<0.001$) or unilateral shoulder ulcer (n=9; $P=0.014$ for albumin, $P=0.021$ for haptoglobin). Ketoprofen did not have a protective effect against shoulder ulcers, but rather appeared to have had a predisposing effect on lactation week 2 (OR 2.70, 95% CI: 1.11-6.56; $P=0.029$). The presence of scars from previous ulcers was the major predisposing factor of the incidence of shoulder ulcers for all lactation weeks ($P<0.001$). The results support the assumption of decreased welfare associated with shoulder ulcers, and imply that in clinical evaluation, especially bilateral shoulder ulcers should be regarded as significant. Further studies are required to find efficient preventative methods for shoulder ulcers and among those, production environment modification should be a priority.

Farm centric and equifinal approach to reduce production diseases on dairy farms

A. Sundrum[1], U. Emanuelson[2], C. Fourichon[3], H. Hogeveen[4], R. Tranter[5] and A. Velarde[6]
[1]UKS, D, 37213 Witzenhausen, Germany, [2]SLU, 75007 Uppsala, Sweden, [3]INRA, 44307 Nantes, France, [4]Wageningen University Livestock Research, Wageningen, the Netherlands, [5]UR, RG6 6AR Reading, United Kingdom, [6]IRTA, 17121 Monells, Spain; sundrum@uni-kassel.de

Negative side effects of the production process on animal health have been discussed since the first ICPD in 1968 and intensive research has been conducted on ways of reducing production diseases (PDs). Nevertheless, dairy farms continue to be plagued by a high prevalence of PDs, adversely affecting productivity, reproduction and animal welfare. Research in animal science has developed many tools under experimental conditions to improve cows' health. However, effectiveness of interventions is generally context-variant and often lacking external validation. An interdisciplinary EU-project (IMPRO) aimed to investigate and promote alternatives to a context-independent handling of tools and measures using a farm centric and equifinal approach to reduce PDs in dairy farming. Equifinal means that the same end state (a low level of selected PDs on the farm level) may be achieved via different paths. Due to the very heterogeneous conditions under which dairy cows are held, generalised recommendations for the implementation of health measures are often both ineffective and inefficient. This results in hindering farmers' readiness to invest in, potentially costly, health measures. Farmers often do not know which measure they should prioritize in order to combat particular problems and which investments could provide an appropriate return of investment. The new alternative approach is based, inter alia, on an impact matrix as a participatory tool (involving farmer, veterinarian and advisor) for: diagnostic work of interactions; evaluation of farm-specific costs; and possible benefits of recommended measures and construction of benchmarks for achievable PD levels. The tool has been created to provide ways of reducing selected PDs (mastitis, metabolic and fertility disorders, and lameness), using particularly data from monthly milk records. The first version of the innovative system-diagnostic tool has been used on 192 farms: 60 in Germany, 23 in Spain, 54 in France, and 55 in Sweden. Conclusions from this exercise were favourable as farmers and their advisors saw the approach as useful. Moreover, results from telephone interviews regarding the uptake of the preventive measures suggested, indicated that 95% of the farmers had implemented one or more of these preventive measures. The feedback from the project was encouraging and provided positive incentives for further development of a farm level diagnostic approach overcoming the faults in previous approaches towards the reduction of PDs on dairy farms.

Refusal to drink in calves in German farms: phenolic compounds a problem?

M. Höltershinken

Clinic for Cattle, University for Veterinary Medicine Hannover, Foundation, Bischofsholer Damm 15, 30173 Hannover, Germany; martin.hoeltershinken@tiho-hannover.de

Since four years, veterinary practices throughout Germany reported problems in cattle populations of various production systems: Calves which had been drinking their colostrum normally on their first day of life quit drinking entirely within the following two days. Their vitality declined and finally they were recumbent. Even intensive clinical care including intravenous rehydratation therapy was unsuccessful. Almost all affected calves died. Scientists of the Clinic for Cattle suspected intoxication with phenolic compounds from grasses (so-called secondary plant substances) in all cases. Thus, blood samples were taken on the second day of life and analyzed for phenols, total protein and gamma-GT. Quantitative photometric analysis of free phenols in serum of these calves was performed. The free phenol compounds were detected by using a sum reaction with Folin-Ciocalteu´s reagent with the variation coefficient being less than 5% for this method. The currently used reference values of 0.26 to 0.42 mmol/l were provided by Hölting. The determination of total protein in serum showed a good ingestion and absorption of colostrum: >50 g/l total protein in serum. In addition, gamma-GT levels in the blood of newborn calves were higher than 250 U/l indicate adequate colostrum quality. The scientists' suspicions were confirmed and increased phenol levels could be shown in affected calves (0.6-1.7 mmol/l). By early separating calves from dams – after having ingested sufficient amounts of colostrum – no later than two days after birth and by feeding milk replacer or milk from cows late in lactation, the disease progress could be stopped in all affected farms. Phenols are compounds with one or several hydroxyl groups attached to a benzene ring. They occur in animals partly through breakdown of aromatic amino acids by intestinal bacteria. However, considerable amounts of phenol-containing compounds are also synthesized in plants. Their functions in a plant range from being pigments to acting as defence substances. Due to the abundance of different molecules in this substance group, a more precise characterization of the molecules responsible for the refusal to drink in calves is currently not possible.

The association between young stock management and antibiotic use in young calves
M. Holstege, A. De Bont-Smolenaars, I. Santman-Berends, G. Witteveen, A. Velthuis and T. Lam
GD Animal Health, Arnsbergstraat 7, 7418 EZ Deventer, the Netherlands;
m.holstege@gdanimalhealth.com

In 2008 the Dutch animal husbandry industry agreed to reduce antimicrobial usage (AMU) with 70% in 2015, relative to the use in 2009. Subsequently, the use of oral antibiotics in calves (0-56 days) on dairy herds has been reduced to a mean animal daily defined dose of antimicrobials per year (DDDAF) of 3.8 in 2014. The median use in this year was 0.0, whereas the variation between herds was large, implicating that there are still farms present with a high AMU (mainly supplied orally) in young calves. To identify factors that were associated with a high AMU, we carried out a study to evaluate whether there is an association between herd management and AMU in dairy and suckler herds in the Netherlands. A case control study was performed in which 200 dairy herds (100 with high AMU in calves between 0-56 days old and 100 with low AMU) and 100 suckler herds (50 with high AMU in calves between 0-56 days old and 50 with low AMU) were selected for participation. Herds with high or low AMU were defined as herds with the 10% highest and lowest antibiotics use during 2012 and 2013. In these herds, a questionnaire was conducted by phone that included questions on general herd management, hygiene, housing, vaccination and calf health. In addition, from these herds routinely collected data on herd size, growth, replacement and the percentage of dead calves was available. Univariable selection was conducted to pre-screen management factors that were potentially associated with AMU status (case or control). Thereafter, a multivariable logistic regression with a logit link function was applied to select the final model using a forward and/or backward selection and elimination method. Confounding was taken into account and the presence of effect modification was checked. Dairy farmers that indicated to start with antimicrobial treatment immediately instead of trying supportive non-antimicrobial treatment first, were classified as case herd 11.4 times more often compared to controls. Other important factors were bedding material used (OR straw combined with slatted floor=4.6), high percentage of respiratory problems (OR=2.3), *Salmonella* status (OR=3.3) and the mindset (OR=4.1) of the farmer. In suckler herds, herd size (OR largest herds=16.4), presence of health problems (OR=4.8), presence of the breed Belgian Blue (OR=13.4) and mindset (OR=8.3) were associated with the case / control status. In this study, factors were identified that characterised herds with structural high AMU in calves (0-56 days old). These factors included both management characteristics and the mindset of the farmer. This information can be used to support farmers to reduce AMU and health problems in calves (0-56 days old).

Monitoring of antimicrobial use and the association with cattle health parameters in the Netherlands

H. Brouwer, I.M.G.A. Santman-Berends, M.A. Gonggrijp, J.J. Hage, A. Smolenaars and G. Van Schaik
GD Animal Health, Arnsbergstraat 7, 7418 EZ Deventer, the Netherlands;
h.brouwer@gdanimalhealth.com

In December 2008, an agreement was reached in the Netherlands to reduce antimicrobial use (AMU) in animal husbandry in order to prevent antimicrobial resistance. A reduction of AMU may require management adjustments from the farmer to maintain a high level of animal health. Since 2011 (veal industry) and 2012 (cattle industry) all antimicrobial supplies, which are a proxy for AMU, to individual cattle farms are registered in a central database. In addition, routinely collected census data about herd size, mortality, fertility, trade, udder and herd health are available for all Dutch cattle herds. Combining these data enabled monitoring of AMU in time and enabled the determination of: (1) associations between AMU and demographic features such as herd size; and (2) associations between AMU and cattle health parameters (CHP) such as BMSCC. Routinely collected data and data of AMU were available for all Dutch cattle herds from January 2011 to July 2014. The routine census data were transformed into CHP and aggregated on herd and quarterly level for five different herd types (i.e. dairy, small-scale, young stock raising, suckling cow and veal calf herds). An annually moving average of the animal daily dose of antibiotic use (DDDAF) was calculated per quarter of the year based on the AMU data. A GEE population-averaged linear, log-linear or logistic regression model was used to evaluate the association between demographic features and AMU and the association between AMU and CHP. The results showed that the median DDDAF was zero in small-scale and young stock raising farms, 2.8 in dairy herds, 0.4 in suckling cow herds and 23.0 in veal calf herds. The median DDDAF decreased from 2011 to 2013 with 24% in veal calf herds and remained stable over time for the other herd types. Herd size and the introduction of cattle on-farm were positively associated with a higher DDDAF in dairy and suckling cow herds. Milk yield was negatively associated with a higher DDDAF in dairy herds. The level of DDDAF was positively associated with cattle mortality on young stock raising, small-scale and veal calf herds. This may indicate that herds with a higher AMU have decreased cattle health. There were an indication that herd management practices differ between dairy herds with high and low AMU as DDDAF was positively associated with the no. of inseminations per cow and negatively associated with the expected time between calvings and BMSCC. This study showed that there is a large variation in AMU between cattle herd types. By regularly analysis of these data, the impact of a further reduction of AMU on cattle health can be monitored.

The relationship between feed intake and cow behaviour

S. Van Der Beek[1], R.M. De Mol[2], R.M.A. Goselink[2] and H.M. Knijn[1]
[1]CRV, Wassenaarweg 20, 6843 NW Arnhem, the Netherlands, [2]Wageningen UR Livestock Research, P.O. Box 338, 6700 AH Wageningen, the Netherlands; sijne.van.der.beek@crv4all.com

One of the most important figures that is still unavailable to dairy farmers is the individual feed intake of their cows. In case a partially mixed ration (PMR) is fed, the individual concentrate intake may be available, but the individual intake at the feeding gate is very variable and still unknown; for a totally mixed ration (TMR), no intake information is available. Individual feed intake can be estimated by cow characteristics and indirect parameters such as parity, milk yield and body weight. These factors can be used to calculate the energy requirements and the predicted feed intake to match these requirements. The difference between the predicted and actual intake may be partially explained by additional measurements of cow behaviour that could be automatically collected by cow sensors, such as rumination activity, eating time or activity. To test this, a dataset of dairy research farm Dairy Campus was used with individual feed intake information measured through a transponder-controlled roughage intake control system (RIC system, Insentec, The Netherlands). The total data set of 2012-2015 included 37,233 cow days with 1,349,368 RIC visits. Cows were equipped with SCR HR tags that detect rumination activity and Nedap Smarttag Leg that detects activity, standing and lying behaviour. Eating time was available through the RIC system: each second a cow was registered in a feeding bin was counted as eating time. Within individual cows, total activity or standing and lying behaviour could not be related to daily dry matter intake. Rumination activity per day also did not correlate well with dry matter intake per day (average $R^2=0.06$). Eating time per day showed a better correlation (average R^2 0.56). For each cow and within each diet or project, medians were calculated for dry matter intake, milk yield, live weight, concentrate intake (in case of PMR), eating time, number of meals and rumination time. These data were analysed by REML to look for factors that may predict dry matter intake. Parity, milk yield and (for PMR) individual concentrate intake will explain up to 63% (PMR) or 79% (TMR) of the variance in dry matter intake; adding live weight will increase these numbers to 70% (PMR) and 81% (TMR). Eating time and rumination time cannot improve these percentages much further; for PMR, the explained variance increases to 73% by adding information on eating time. The main determinants of feed intake thus remain to be parity, milk yield and live weight. Eating time, rumination time and activity may be used for individual cow management, but are with our current information difficult to use as predictors of dry matter intake in general.

A new endoscopic approach for bronchoalveolar lavage at cattle-for better results in BRD diagnostics

W. Hasseler[1] and F. Schlederer[2]
[1]*Private Practice, Waldstrasse 8, 26871 Papenburg, Germany,* [2]*Private Pracitce, Lichtegg 1, 4770 Andorf, Austria; fam-hasseler@t-online.de*

Bronchoalveolar lavage (BAL) is a very common and useful diagnostic approach for bovine respiratory disease (BRD) management. Traditionally the lavage is carried out through the trachea (trans tracheal lavage; TTL). A new hand held multiscope (endoscope with several different functions; Ivetscope, Quidee, Germany) has been designed for a more convenient way of BAL under field conditions. The aim of this study was to compare two different methods of BAL – the puncture of the trachea with the transtracheal lavage against the oro-laryngeal methode. The new endoscope approach was applied on 64 calves (age 2-22 weeks) with bovine respiratory disease (BRD) history. Bronchoalveolar liquid was sampled for microbial and virological evaluation. 32 calves were collected by the traditional way (TTL), whereas 32 calves were examined by the use of this new endoscope (BAL). The pistol-shaped, hand-held and cordless endoscope, reaches 40 cm in length, with 2 working tunnels. A camera is positioned next to the corpus, so that a visual adspection can be carried out simultaneously. Calves were sedated (xylazine, 0.2 mg/kg) prior to treatment, kept into sterno-ventral position with the head held manually by the farmer. Each time two samples of broncho-alveolar liquid were collected: From the deeper part of the lung (>50 cm distance) and from the upper part of the bronchus (30-40 cm). They were split equally into a modified New York City medium (NYC medium; Biocheck) and a sterile vessel for further examination. On average in a total of 15.4% of all cases no agent could be identified. With this new method only in 6.1% (4 times less!) of all cases the responsible microbiological cause could not be identified, whereas the traditional technique reveals 25% 'no agents' ($P<0.01$). Single strains of bacteria/virus results were obtained two times more often with the BAL method (60.6 vs 34.4%) than with the TTL approach. BRSV was found in total of 9,2% of all analysed samples, with no difference between the two methods. *Mycoplasma bovis* was found three times more often (33.3 vs 9.4%) with the endoscope lavage (BAL). *Pasteurella multocida* was the most single prominent bacteria to be found in the lung, in total 9.2%. 15.6% of all cases monocausal cases are diagnosed with *P. multocida* by TAL vs 3.0% by BAL; whereas BAL revealed *P. multocida/M. bovis* 5 times more often than with the TAL method (15.2 vs 3.1%). The new BAL method with the Ivetscope seems to result in an obviously more precise identification of relevant respiratory tract bacteria. *M. bovis* might be more difficult to collect in traditional TTL and could be overgrown by other bacteria as the mixed infection and contamination rate is significantly higher in TTL sampling.

Effects of herd health management on animal health in organic dairy herds in Sweden

K. Sjöström and U. Emanuelson
Swedish University of Agricultural Sciences, Department of Clinical Sciences, P.O. Box 7054,
75007 Uppsala, Sweden; karin.sjostrom@slu.se

Production diseases are a major issue for dairy herds, with implications on the welfare of the animals and on the farm economy. A high standard of animal health and welfare is an important aspect of organic dairy production and an important incentive to the consumers to buy organic products. One of the major aims of the IMPRO project (impro-dairy.eu), of which this study is a part of, was to design farm-specific animal health plans and proactive monitoring and prevention protocols. The objective of this study was to assess potential effects on the general health of Swedish organic dairy herds by applying these tools. In this study there were three groups of farms. In farms in group 1 (G1, n=32) management measures, as part of an animal health plan, were identified using a participatory process, involving the farmer, a veterinarian and / or an advisor and a researcher and applying an Impact Matrix analysis. In farms in group 2 (G2, n=21) the participatory process was followed by applying a farm-specific pro-active monitoring and preventive approach during the following year. Finally, a control group (CG, n=52) of farms were included in this study, where no actions were taken within the project. The general health of the herds was assessed by the Swedish 'Animal Welfare Signals' (AWS) from the fiscal years 2012, prior to any actions, and 2014, during and / or after the actions on the farms. Differences between groups of farms prior to the actions were assessed by Kruskal-Wallis tests, while differences between the groups in the change from 2012 to 2014 were assessed by analysis of variance. The median herd size was 73, 77, and 61 cows, in G1, G2 and CG, respectively, while median kg milk production per cow and year was 9242, 9000 and 8884. There were no statistically significant differences in the selected AWS between the groups of herds in 2012. Herds in G2 had a significantly reduced 24 h calf mortality rate, compared to the other groups, and also a significantly reduced rate of veterinary treated diseases, while there were no differences in terms of on-farm cow mortality, culling, veterinary treated cases of mastitis, or bulk tank milk somatic cell counts. Our results indicate that the more complete, and longitudinal, approach to herd health management was beneficial, but the results need to be verified with a longer period of follow-up. This project has received funding from the European Union's Seventh Framework Programme for research, technological development and demonstration under grant agreement n° 311824 (IMPRO).

Reticular pH as a means of diagnosing subacute ruminal acidosis (SARA) in periparturient cows

S. Sato[1], Y. Watanabe[1], T. Ichijo[1], M. Maeda[2] and H. Yano[2]
[1]Iwate University, Cooperative Department of Veterinary Medicine, Morioka, Iwate, 020-8550, Japan, [2]NOSAI Yamagata, Mogami Veterinary Clinical Center, Shinjo, Yamagata, 996-0051, Japan; sshigeru@iwate-u.ac.jp

Reticular and ruminal pH levels are positively correlated, and subacute ruminal acidosis (SARA) has been diagnosed using reticular pH levels in experimental cows. However, few studies have described the potential of measuring reticular pH for diagnosing SARA in periparturient cows. Therefore, we aimed to assess the rate of SARA incidence in periparturient cows under field conditions to determine whether SARA can be diagnosed using reticular pH levels. In a preliminary experiment run four times, eight rumen-cannulated Holstein steers were fed hay or a SARA-inducing diet for 7 days. Wireless radio-transmission pH-sensors (YCOW-S; DKK-Toa, Yamagata, Japan) were placed in the ventral sac of the rumen and the reticulum of each individual, and pH was measured every 10 minutes. We obtained final data from 28 individuals steers over 56 days, and divided cattle into SARA and non-SARA groups using the more commonly used ruminal pH. Individuals with a ruminal pH of <5.6 for >3 hr per day were placed in the SARA group. Individuals with SARA showed a mean reticular pH of 6.1 over a 24-hr period, a mean difference of 0.7 among days, and decreases of 0.4 and 0.6 from the maximum value for two and three hrs per day. We then used 29 cows from six herds for a field experiment. We measured the reticular pH during the periparturient period, and estimated the rate of SARA incidence from the day to 28 days after parturition using the diagnostic information obtained in the preliminary experiment. The 24-hr mean reticular pH of periparturient cows in healthy herds was stable, but values fluctuated markedly in pre- and post-parturition cows and differed among individuals in SARA herds. Using the 24-hr mean reticular pH as a diagnostic tool (i.e. a pH of <6.1), SARA was found in 22 of 29 post-parturition cows (75.9%) and in 244 of 736 (33.2%) total individuals across all estimated days. Using a ruminal pH of <5.6 for >3 hr per day, we diagnosed SARA in 171 of 244 (70.1%) cows in the SARA group and 9 of 492 (1.8%) cows in the non-SARA group. Similarly, using among-day variance, and decreases of 0.4 and 0.6 from maximum values in reticular pH, SARA was diagnosed in 74.2%, 23.3% and 13.8% of total individuals across all estimated days, respectively. We conclude that reticular pH can diagnose SARA in periparturient cows with relative accuracy. Specifically, the 24-hr mean (6.1), among-day variance (0.7), and decreases from the maximum value for 2 and 3 hr per day (0.4 and 0.6) are useful diagnostic tools.

Improvement in the capabilities of a wireless transmission pH measuring system

H. Mizuguchi[1], N. Kakizaki[1], K. Ito[1], D. Kishi[1] and S. Sato[2]
[1]DKK-Toa Yamagata Co, R&D Department, 711-109, Aza-Fukudayama, Oaza-Fukuda, Shinjyo-shi, yamagata, 996-0053, Japan, [2]Iwate University, Cooperative Department of Veterinary Medicine, Faculty of Agriculture, 3-18-8 Ueda, Morioka-shi, Iwate 020-8550, Japan; mizuguchi@toadkk.co.jp

The prototype of a wireless transmission pH measurement system for fluid in the rumen was reported previously at the 14th ICPD in 2010. Briefly, the system consisted of a wireless pH sensor, a data measurement receiver, a relay unit, and a personal computer installed with special software. The maximum data transmission distance of the prototype was from 20-30 meters, and missing data were frequent occurrences (missed rate=10-15% of the total transmitted data). Further, the prototype software simply received the data, which were regularly displayed and saved on a personal computer. Improvements to the data transmission system were required due to the high missing data rate of the prototype. The purpose of this study was to decrease the missing data rate and to improve the utilization of transmitted data. The capabilities of the wireless transmission pH measurement system were improved. To reduce missing data,we experimentally evaluated the performance of several types of antenna and developed a high-performance antenna. As a result, electric field strength was improved from -98±5 (M±SD, n=6, at 20 m distance from sensor) dBm in the prototype to -78±5 dBm, after the improvement. In addition, the pH sensor device and software were improved. If datatransmission conditions were unstable, the pH sensor device temporarily saved the data (up to 400 of data), and the saved data were then transmitted automatically to a personal computer when transmission conditions stabilized. As a result, the phenomenon that data disappeared was improved. The data disappeared was 00.0±0.0% (n=6). The improved software automatically displayed charts and analyzed data features, further improving its utilization. Consequently, the improved wireless transmission pH measurement system dramatically reduced the missing data rate and all data were efficiently received by a personal computer. Due to the improvement of the transmission system, the battery life of the sensor device was considerably extended, up to 90-120 days, through a reduction of the retry number of attempted transmissions. The improved wireless transmission pH measurement system consisting of an improved, high-performance antenna, a data storage function(on the sensor device),and automatically operated simplified software would make possible effective utilization of pH data for analysis.

Evaluation of a new portable blood cow side test for calcium

M. Neumayer[1] and H. Hilmert[2]
[1]KIM private consultancy, Hanselmannsiedlung 227, 5741 Neukirchen am Großvenediger, Austria, [2]Institute for bovine medicine, Veterinary University of Berliin, Königsweg 65, 14163 Berlin, Germany; neumayer.tierarzt@sbg.at

Cows around calving are very vulnerable and susceptible for any metabolic disturbances. To identify cows at risk for hypocalcemia, a new portable on farm photometer was developed. Thus enabling the vet to make on farm cow side wise decisions. The aim was to evaluate this new cow side test for calcium measurements. A new hand held photometer (Vetphotometer, quidee.com) was designed for farm evaluations on cows at risk for the major problem areas of dairy cows (fat mobilization, hypocalcemia and hypomagnesemia) or to serve as a prognostic parameter for successful surgical interventions (l-lactate). Two studies have therefore been conducted to prove the accuracy of this new tool for calcium measurements. In this first study, 20 heparinized blood samples from lactating cows have been submitted to 2 different testing photometer protocols. The trial group was evaluated by the vetphotometer at 520 nm with modified detergent (Diaglobal) and compared to the results obtained by spectral photometric evaluations (Spectral photometer LS 500; 578 nm), which are regarded as 'golden standard'. In a second study, 15 heparinized blood samples from Holstein cows were collected for calcium measurements run either by Solaar AAS (Atomic Absorption Spectrophotometry; Thermo Fisher) or by the digital Vetphotometer. In the first study, a very high correlation between the two different photometric calcium measurements was obtained. A linear correlation of 0.9717x + 0.0152 mmol/l was achieved. In the second trial a linear correlation of 0.9476 of total calcium between the two methods was achieved. A new digital calcium cow side approach showed a high correlation and accuracy compared to standard laboratory analyses. Therefore, it can be concluded that this new approach serves very well as a quick testing for calcium in the blood plasma of lactating cows to help better estimate the need for suitable treatment and feeding management decisions. Monitoring calcium levels in dairy cows can be done very easily and quick cow side wise.

Connection between biochemical blood indicators of calcium metabolism and BCS

J. Starič, M. Klinkon, M. Nemec and J. Ježek
University of Ljubljana, Veterinary faculty, Gerbičeva 60, 1000 Ljubljana, Slovenia;
joze.staric@vf.uni-lj.si

Body condition score (BCS) is a well-known factor in etiology of negative energy balance (NEB) and periparturient hypocalcaemia. In a present study we wanted to test in farm settings influence of BCS on total blood serum calcium (Ca), inorganic phosphate (iP), bone alkaline phosphatase (bALP) and C-terminal telopetide of collagen I (CTx) in 20 healthy multiparous Holstein Friesian dairy cows. Cows were sampled and BCS assessed 4 times: 1. at early dry period (1 month before calving), 2. close up dry period (10 or less days before calving), 3. early fresh (within 48 h after calving) and 4. 10 to 20 days in milk, during winter time, when cows were kept indoors in loose housing system with cubicles. The mean BCS in the tested group of cows was 3.35 (range 2.50 to 5.00). Mean Ca concentrations were 2.32, 2.15, 1.81 and 2.24 mmol/l in 1., 2., 3. and 4. sampling respectively. Mean iP concentrations were 2.14, 1.88, 1.51 and 2.05 mmol/l in 1., 2., 3. and 4. sampling respectively. Mean bALP activities were 15.38, 16.93, 31.01 and 24.26 U/l in 1., 2., 3. and 4. sampling respectively. Mean CTx concentrations were 0.22, 0.14, 0.62 and 1.18 ng/ml in 1., 2., 3. and 4. sampling respectively. We noticed a weak positive correlation between BCS and CTx (τ=0.33, P=0.054) just at early dry period. No other significant correlations between BCS and measured parameters of bone metabolism were noticed in other sampling times. CTx is a bone resorption marker and positive correlation with BCS could be explained by lower feed consumption resulting in lower Ca intake than needed for maintenance and foetal growth. Negative Ca balance activated bone resorption which resulted in increase in CTx in cows with higher BCS. To proof this assumption studies with more cows are needed. The importance of BCS in bone metabolism of dairy cows is highly suggestive in this study and thus should be an important point of any dairy herd health programme.

Evaluation of levels of Ca, free triiodothyronine, free thyroxine and insulin in cows with ketosis

S. Kozat

Yuzuncu Yıl University, Faculty of Veterinary Medicine, Internal of Medicine, Tuşba-Van, 65010, Turkey; skozat@hotmail.com

The aim of this study was to evaluate thyroid, insulin hormones, and calcium levels in cows with subclinical and clinical ketosis. The study included twelve cows with clinical ketosis, eight cows with subclinical ketosis and ten healthy cows. Before treatment, serum glucose, calcium, free triiodothyronine (fT3), and free thyroxine (fT4) levels in cows with subclinical ketosis have been found lower than control group ($P<0.001$, $P<0.01$; $P<0.01$ and $P<0.001$, respectively) and plasma BHBA levels in cows with subclinical ketosis were higher than control group ($P<0.001$). Before treatment, plasma BHBA concentrations in cows with clinical ketosis have been found higher than control group ($P<0.001$). Serum glucose, calcium, fT3 and fT4 levels have been found lower than control group ($P<0.001$, $P<0.01$, $P<0.001$, and $P<0.001$, respectively). At the 3rd day after treatment; while plasma BHBA concentration in cows with clinical ketosis has been reached to normal level ($P>0.05$), glucose level has increased, however it has been found lower than control group ($P<0.001$). Although serum calcium, fT3, and fT4 levels have increased; their levels have been found lower than control group ($P<0.05$, $P<0.01$, and $P<0.001$, respectively). Significant changes in calcium, free T3 and T4 have been determined in groups with both subclinical and clinical ketosis. It is concluded that treatment by considering levels of insulin and calcium will increase the effect of treatment along with prognosis.

Impact of fatty acid supplementation on basal adenosine triphosphate release from bovine erythrocyte

D. Revskij[1], S. Haubold[1], T. Viergutz[1], C. Weber[1], A. Tuchscherer[1], A. Tröscher[2], H.J. Schuberth[3], H.M. Hammon[1] and M. Mielenz[1]
[1]Leibniz Institute for Farm Animal Biology (FBN), Wilhelm-Stahl-Allee 2, 18196 Dummerstorf, Germany, [2]BASF SE, Chemiestraße 22, 68623 Lampertheim, Germany, [3]University of Veterinary Medicine Hannover, Bischofsholer Damm 15, 30173 Hannover, Germany; revskij@fbn-dummerstorf.de

Red blood cells (RBC) have been shown to release adenosine triphosphate (ATP) in response to physiological stimuli like mechanical deformation. The signaling mechanism of ATP release involves several membrane associated proteins and allows RBC to participate in the control of vascular caliber and thus may affect energy partitioning. In addition, extracellular ATP can also act as an immunomodulator. It has been shown that the intake of fatty acids (FA) influence membrane composition of incorporated FA. Common diets in dairy production are often based on corn silage that deliver lower amounts of essential n-3 polyunsaturated fatty acids as α-linolenic acid (ALA) compared to pasture based systems, and also results in less ruminal conjugated linoleic acids (CLA) synthesis. The aim of this study was to evaluate the effect of a diet low in ALA content, followed by essential FA and/or CLA supplementation on the basal ATP release from bovine RBC. Four rumen fistulated German Holstein cows (18 weeks in milk at start of the study) were arranged in a 4×4 Latin square model. Cows were fed a total mixed ration based on corn silage (6.8 MJ NEL/kg of dry matter) and supplemented by abomasal administration twice per day with three successively increased lipid dosages, each dosage was given for 2 weeks, followed by a three week wash out phase. Supplements were coconut oil (Sanct Bernhard) (CO; 38, 77 and 153 g/d), linseed-safflower oil mix (Derby® linseed oil, Gefro® safflower oil), delivering essential FA (EFA; 42, 82 and 163 g/d), Lutalin® (BASF) (CLA; c9,t11 and t10,c12 in equal amounts; 16, 32 and 64 g/d) or both (EFA; 42, 82 and 163 g/d + CLA; 16, 32 and 64 g/d). From whole blood samples RBC were isolated at the end of each supplementation and wash out period and diluted to a hematocrit of 0.04%, 0.02% and 0.01%. The basal ATP release was measured by the luciferin-luciferase technique. ATP release was normalized 10^8 cells. Data were analysed by mixed model of SAS using repeated measurement analysis with week in milk as covariate. Basal ATP release was increased by the supplementation of CO, CLA, EFA and the combination of CLA and EFA compared to the wash out periods ($P<0.05$). Our results suggest that a supplementation of an additional energy source, i.e. FA influence capillary caliber via ATP release and may improve energy partitioning. Further studies should be focused on the regulatory mechanisms of ATP release in bovine RBCs.

A new and simple methode to deal with teat injuries

F. Schlederer
Private Practice, Lichtegg 1, 4770 Lichtegg, Austria; vet.lichtegg@speed.at

Teat injuries are common in dairy cattle, around 2-3% are affected. They can be divided into two categories (external or internal injuries). They often result in premature culling of affected cows. Surgery and treatment of these injuries has been described and discussed intensively. However the question whether complete rest (no milking) or temporary resting of the injured teat by temporary cessation of milking or continuous milking is not yet clearly answered and may vary from case to case. This paper describes a new technique that allows a permanent milk flow alongside an undisturbed healing process of all types of teat injuries. Cows with covered or open teat injuries are suitable to benefit from the permanent milk flow system. A silicon-like catheter (TEATflow) has been designed for that purpose. The described surgery of open lesions as well differs from traditional methods as no blood stasis is applied. Prior to intervention Oxytocin (10 I.U.) is administered intravenously to achieve an intensive milk drop down. Single suture knots are carried out to achieve only a slight, but careful wound closure. This procedure is aimed to result in a faster consolidation of fibrocytes for a undisturbed healing process. To avoid any internal milk teat pressure, that might disturb the accumulation of fibrocytes, milk is allowed to permanently exit the teat by the inserted catheter for 9 consecutive days. The insertion is eased by application with the help of the traditional Fuerstenberg-catheter. Penethamat-Penicillin (2×5 Mio I.E./day i.m.) is administered systemically to reduce concurrent teat infections. No further local antibiotic treatment is applied. Nine individual cow case studies are reported. Occurence of clinical mastitis, restoration of complete milkability and evolution of somatic cell count (prior and around eight weeks after treatment) are documented as potential success criteria. The mean somatic cell count of all cows was 140,000/ml prior to treatment. All cows fully restored milkability. One cow was infected by a clinical mastitis, which reflects a mastitis infection risk of 11%. The mean somatic cell count (SCC) at eight weeks after surgery was 67,500/ml, which reflects a 19% increase of prior SCC. Due to the limited numbers this is not statistically significant. Six cows showed an augmented SCC, whereas 3 cows revealed a reduced SCC. The new treatment and surgery method for all type of teat lesions offers a very practical, simple and easy way to successfully regain milkability. As the risk for clinical mastitis seems lower than reported elsewhere, the permanent milk flow system obviously seems to allow a faster and complete healing process at a very low infection risk due to the permanent open teat canal with consistent flushing.

Reduced ivermectin efficacy against *Ostertagia* in a Dutch cattle herd
M. Holzhauer, C. Hegeman and D. Van Doorn
GD Deventer, P.O. Box 9, 7400 AA Deventer, the Netherlands; m.holzhauer@gddiergezondheid.nl

Gastro-intestinal parasitic infections in cattle result in aspecific symptoms, like growth retardation, etc. Infections with gastro intestinal nematodes (GIN) regularly resulted in major problems in young stock, but is limited in most young stock in Western Europe nowadays. The most recent inventory about management measures and anthelmintic usage for the control of GIN infections in the Netherlands was conducted in 2010. In this study, an indication for resistance to macrocyclic lactones (ML; applied per injection) in Coöperia spp. was found. In Europe, resistance to ML in cattle has been described several times. In June 2015, a fattening bull of 1.5 years was offered at the Dutch Animal Health (GD) for pathological examination. The bull was purchased on 16 April 2015, treated with an ivermectin pour-on and pastured without delay. In the previous year, the bulls were also on pasture and were treated with eprinomectin pour-on at the time of housing. A remarkably high number of strongyle type eggs (1000 eggs per gram faeces (epg)) was observed in the post mortem investigated bull. This was noteworthy because of the bulls age and the history of treatment. To rule out under dosing by the farmer and to investigate the possibility of reduced efficacy of an ivermectin pour-on on GIN, an additional treatment under supervision of a GD-veterinarian combined with examination of faecal samples was conducted. The pilot, performed in the period June-July 2015, consisted of the following components: rectally taken manure samples collected from bulls, epg counts faeces and differentiation of cultured larvae, application of pour-on at 4 bulls, rectal taken faecal samples from the same bulls, epg counts, larval cultures and differentiation and faecal egg count reduction test (FCERT). The samples were examined individually at the GD laboratory using the modified McMaster method. FCERT was used to demonstrate a change in the reduction in anthelmintic efficacy as described previously. The guidelines of WAAVP, define anthelmintic resistance as present if the percentage reduction in egg count is less than 95%. The FECRT based on EPGs was 65% ($100 \times (1-(102/288))$) and so indicates a reduced efficacy. However the number of sampled and treated animals (6) was lower than within the guidelines of WAAVP (10 animals). Under ideal circumstances we would have tested more animals, but in this herd that was not possible. The strongyle larvae were all determined as *Ostertagia ostertagi* and a single *Strongyloides*. The set-up of the pilot experiment did not allow for a discrimination between reduced efficacy of the active ML ingredient and reduced efficacy due to the method of application. Unfortunately, a repeat experiment using a different application route of the ML was not possible in this herd.

Animal health management in Burgers' Zoo

C. Mager
Royal Burgers' Zoo, Antoon van Hooffplein 1, 6816 SH Arnhem, the Netherlands;
events@burgerszoo.nl

Constanze Mager is zoologist and head of education of Royal Burgers' Zoo. Next to her core tasks, she also coordinates most of the scientific research done in Burgers' Zoo and is busy in promoting nature conservation. Naturally, she will tell the participants about the groundbreaking non-invasive behavioral research that has been done in the zoo on great apes in the past. Also, she will give a few examples of the most recent research projects. But above all, during her speech at Burgers' Zoo, Constanze will take you on a virtual journey through the zoo, while addressing all the sessions' main themes of the last three conference days. This way, we will recap some topics from a totally different view, as it is now all about zoo related issues and tropical animals. A few examples: managing exotic animals means of course being very careful with the temperature and humidity of their environment. Burgers' Bush, a rainforest hall as large as 1.5 soccer fields, is a good example. But also extremely important is the prevention of heat stress in antelopes when the animals are transferred to another zoo. When it comes to gut health, the spectacled langurs are a nice example in the zoo. These leaf-eating primates have a ruminant-like stomach, without being ruminants. Just since the last few years we get more and more knowledge how to optimize these delicate monkeys' diet, in order to keep their stomachs' microbiota on a good level. Lactation seems the most natural thing in mammals, but even wild animals in human care might have trouble with it. Learn more about the supported lactation in our zoo's aardvarks. And did you know that a German veterinary specialist team travels all around Europe to check fertility problems in elephants, rhinos and bears?

Authors index

A

Abdalla, H. — 123
Abeni, F. — 83
Albaaj, A. — 160
Alizadeh, A.R. — 111
Alkan, A. — 171
Allaart, J. — 64
Alsaaod, M. — 32, 33, 44
Amaefule, B.C. — 92
Ampe, B. — 38, 89
Antanaitis, R. — 168
Araujo, M. — 115
Arne, A. — 73
Aschenbroich, R. — 61
Azem, E. — 110

B

Babiker, S. — 123
Badiei, K. — 106, 121
Bailey, R.A. — 142
Baling, P. — 98
Balli, B. — 127
Bareille, N. — 181
Barrow, P. — 156
Batmaz, H. — 138, 139
Baulain, U. — 49
Baxter, E.M. — 173
Bee, G. — 67
Beer, G. — 33, 44
Beineke, A. — 53
Bell, N. — 31
Benedictus, L. — 101
Bennett, R.M. — 148
Benson, J. — 62
Benthem De Grave, X. — 166
Bernardeau, M. — 62
Berri, M. — 77
Bestman, M. — 48
Biemans, F. — 35
Bijma, P. — 35
Binnendijk, G.P. — 39, 40
Bisgaard, M. — 140, 141
Blake3, D.P. — 142
Blakeley, W. — 151
Blanco-Penedo, I. — 181

Boerhout, E.M. — 101
Bogado Pascottini, O. — 157
Bolhuis, J.E. — 66, 165, 174, 177
Bollwein, H. — 98
Bonny, P. — 41
Borchardt, S. — 100
Borgijink, S. — 65
Bos, E.-J. — 38
Bossers, A. — 65
Boudon, A. — 144
Boyle, L.A. — 37, 129, 130, 131
Bracke, M.B.M. — 179
Brenninkmeyer, C. — 48
Breves, G. — 110, 114
Brooshooft, S.D. — 175
Brouwer, H. — 34, 189
Bruckmaier, R.M. — 93, 99, 102, 104, 108, 111, 118, 119, 158
Bussy, F. — 77

C

Calderon-Diaz, J. — 131
Camacho, J. — 103
Campos, P.H.R.F. — 78
Canibe, N. — 58
Cantaloube, E. — 144
Carp-Van Dijken, S. — 116
Celebi, D. — 45
Cengiz, M. — 127
Cengiz, S. — 127
Chalmeh, A. — 106, 121
Chamorro, S. — 88
Chatelet, A. — 145
Chaussé, A.M. — 156
Chen, J. — 97, 104, 105, 158
Christensen, H. — 140, 141
Christensen, J.P. — 140, 141
Chuppava, B. — 56
Clark, A. — 146
Cohrs, I. — 110
Cools, A. — 143
Counotte, G.H.M. — 112

D

Daemen, A.J.J.M. — 101

Dame-Korevaar, M.A.	52	Eisenberg, S.W.F.	101
Dänicke, S.	94	Eising, I.	42
Da Silva, C.L.A.	164	Elbawab, I.	172
Davidek, J.	82	Elbehiry, M.	172
Dawn, C.	69	Emanuelson, U.	159, 181, 186, 192
De Bont-Smolenaars, A.	188	Engberg, R.M.	58
De Bree, F.M.	65	Engels, A.	51
De Bruijn, C.	64	Ersoz, U.	45
De Bruijn, N.	65	Eusemann, B.K.	49
De Gouw, P.	182	Evans, T.J.	161
De Greeff, A.	64	Ezeokonkwo, M.C.	92
Degroote, J.	75, 79, 87		
De Jong, E.	41	**F**	
De Jong, I.C.	47, 175, 182	Fabri, T.	65
De Jong, M.C.M.	35	Farci, F.	134
Dekkers, J.C.M.	150	Farquhar, R.	146
De Koeijer, A.A.	163	Farzan, V.	135
De Koning, D.B.	120, 164	Feldmann, M.	98
De Koster, J.	96	Ferrante, V.	48
Delago, F.	62	Fievez, V.	117
De Lange, C.F.M.	135	Fischer, E.A.J.	52
De Los Mozos, J.	50	Forte, C.	63
Demais, H.	77	Foster, N.	156
Demeyer, D.	147	Foucras, G.	160
Demko, G.	151	Fourichon, C.	181, 186
De Mol, R.M.	190	Fujii, N.	167
Den Uijl, I.E.M.	116		
De Smet, S.	63, 75, 79, 87	**G**	
De Vries Reilingh, G.	104	Galbraith, E.	62
Dewulf, J.	147	Galli, A.	83
Diana, A.	131	Gandy, J.	95
Dijkman, R.	43	García-Ruiz, A.I.	50, 88
Dijkstra, J.	102	García Suárez, M.	77
Dijkstra, T.	34	Gaughan, J.B.	80
Dirx, N.	177	Gerrits, W.J.J.	132
Djemali, M.	85	Ghorbani, A.	111
Dogan, E.	45	Gibbs, K.	62
Doroshchuk, S.	91	Gilbert, H.	145
Doyle, B.	129, 130	Giles, T.	156
Drevinskas, T.	153	Girard, M.	67
Dunkelberger, J.R.	150	Gocsik, E.	124, 126, 175
Dūrītis, I.	68	Golian, A.	79, 87
Duval, J.E.	181	Gondret, F.	145, 155
		Gonggrijp, M.A.	36, 43, 189
E		Goselink, R.M.A.	39, 40, 190
Edwards, S.A.	173	Granz, S.	159
Eisa, N.	123	Grigonis, A.	168

Groot Koerkamp, P.W.G. 174
Gross, J.J. 99, 102, 104, 108, 118, 119
Guan, X. 70
Gumen, A. 171
Gunnarsson, S. 48, 180
Gunnink, H. 182
Günther, R. 51
Gutzwiller, A. 67

H

Hage, J.J. 189
Hallén Sandgren, C. 159
Hamali, H. 170
Hammon, H.M. 107, 198
Hamrouni, A. 85
Hanlon, A. 129, 130
Häsler, B. 134
Hassaneen, A.S.A. 167
Hasseler, W. 191
Haubold, S. 198
Hausegger, T. 32
Hayirli, A. 45, 127
Heerkens, J.L.T. 48
Hegeman, C. 200
Heidari, M. 90
Heinonen, M. 149
Heinzl, I. 61, 74
Hendriks, W.H. 71
Herdt, T.H. 95
Hering, S. 154
Hernández-Castellano, L.E. 93
Hernandez, L.L. 93
Hetchler, B.P. 81
Heuermann, A. 54
Heuwieser, W. 84, 86, 100
Hilbrands, A.M. 81
Hilmert, H. 195
Hinrichsen, L.K. 48
Hipp, M. 169
Hira, F. 127
Hogeveen, H. 122, 186
Hojberg, O. 58
Holstege, M. 188
Höltershinken, M. 187
Holzhauer, M. 36, 43, 200
Hoofs, A. 177
Hoste, H. 71

Hostens, M. 117, 157
Hovinen, M. 133
Huber, K. 94
Hulme, S. 156
Hussein, F. 172

I

Ichijo, T. 193
Ieda, N. 167
Ilgaza, A. 73
Ilves, A. 108
Inoue, N. 167
Ipharraguerre, I.R. 69
Ito, K. 194

J

Jaakson, H. 108
Jackisch, T. 54
Jacobson, L.D. 81
Jacobs, V. 115
Jansman, A.J.M. 60, 65, 132
Janssens, G. 38
Jensen, B.B. 58
Ježek, J. 196
Johnston, L.J. 81
Jones, P.J. 148
Jorjong, S. 117
Junker, K. 43

K

Kakizaki, N. 194
Kalkowska, D.A. 163
Kamphues, J. 53, 54, 55, 57
Kampman-Van De Hoek, E. 132
Karakaya, E. 171
Karhapää, M. 144
Karis, P. 108
Karpovaitė, A. 153
Kaske, M. 98
Kato, M. 167
Keller, B. 56
Kemp, B. 66, 97, 102, 104, 105, 120, 158, 164, 174, 176
Kenéz, Á. 94
Kerrigan, M.A. 150
Keskin, A. 171
Kessler, E.C. 118

Kienberger, H.	107	Loisel, F.	152
Kimura, K.	167	Lorenzo, E.	147
Kishi, D.	194	Lucy, M.C.	161
Klinger, S.	114	Lunney, J.K.	150
Klinkenberg, M.	147		
Klinkon, M.	196	**M**	
Kluivers-Poodt, M.	177	Madouasse, A.	181
Knijn, H.M.	190	Maeda, M.	193
Knol, E.F.	164	Maeda, Y.	137
Koets, A.P.	101	Maes, D.	38, 147
Kohler, P.	33	Mager, C.	201
Kok, A.	97, 105	Mahmoud, M.	178
Kolisek, M.	154	Mahrt, A.	100
Kölln, M.	54, 57	Majdeddin, M.	79, 87
König, S.	178	Mangelinckx, S.	63
Korbel, R.	46	Manoj, T.	72
Kortes, H.E.	124	Manzanilla, E.G.	130, 131
Kozat, S.	197	Marchewka, J.	37
Kredel, R.	32	Marey, M.	172
Krieger, M.	181	Maruška, A.	153
Krupa, E.	128	Matsuda, F.	167
Krupová, Z.	128	Matsuyama, S.	167
Kubilienė, L.	153	Mayasari, N.	97, 104
Kushibiki, S.	137	Ma, Z.	75
Kyriazakis, I.	142, 146, 152	McElroy, M.	131
		McGettrick, S.	131
L		Mecitoglu, Z.	139
Lambrecht, J.	62	Mee, J.F.	37
Lammers, A.	176	Mehrvar, N.	170
Lam, T.J.G.M.	102, 116, 188	Mengistu, G.	71
Lannoo, F.	117	Merckx, W.	143
Laurenssen, B.F.A.	164, 165	Mereu, A.	69
Lauridsen, C.	58	Merlot, E.	145, 155
Laurila, T.	149	Metwally, K.	172
Lauwaerts, A.	143	Meunier-Salaün, M.C.	144
Lees, A.M.	80	Mevius, D.J.	52
Lees, J.C.	80	Mica, J.	50, 88
Le Floc'h, N.	78, 144, 145, 152, 155, 156	Michaličková, M.	128
Leibfacher, C.	51	Michiels, J.	63, 75, 79, 87
Leijten, F.	182	Mickienė, R.	153
Lelešius, R.	153	Mielenz, M.	198
Leonard, F.C.	131	Miersch, C.	154
Lewis, C.R.G.	146	Millet, S.	38
Liepa, L.	68, 184	Minabe, S.	167
Lietz, G.	142, 146	Mirzaei, A.	121
Ling, K.	108	Misu, R.	167
Loi-Brügger, A.	57	Mizuguchi, H.	194

Modaresi, M. 90
Mohamadi, M. 106
Molist, F. 70, 166
Momenifar, F. 106
Montagne, L. 152
Montalvo, G. 147
Moons, C.P.H. 89
Moor, C.D. 143
Moriarty, J. 131
Mulder, H.A. 164
Müller, H. 33

N

Naguib, M. 176
Naniwa, Y. 167
Navarro-Villa, A. 50
Nejat Dehkordi, S. 125
Nemec, M. 196
Neumayer, M. 195
Niederhauser, J. 44
Niederwerder, M. 150
Niemi, J.K. 148, 149
Nikitkina, E. 91
Niozas, G. 98
Nishimura, K. 137
Noblet, J. 78
Nolan, M.J. 142
Norby, B. 95
Norring, M. 133
Nystén, M. 185
Nyvall Collen, P. 77

O

Ohkura, S. 167
Oikeh, I. 142
Oishi, S. 167
Okumus, Z. 45
Oliviero, C. 149
Olsen, R.H. 140, 141
Opsomer, G. 96, 109, 117, 157
Orro, T. 185
Ots, M. 108
Oude Lansink, A.G.J.M. 124, 126
Ouweltjes, W. 39, 40
Ovyn, A. 63, 79
Oxley, A. 142

P

Palme, R. 89
Papasolomontos, S. 140
Parmentier, H.K. 104
Pärn, P. 108
Pastor, J.J. 69
Pearce, P. 151
Pellikaan, W.F. 71
Peltoniemi, O. 185
Petow, S. 49
Petzl, W. 169
Pieper, R. 59
Pierre, M. 109
Piñeiro, C. 147
Poock, S.E. 161
Pors, S.E. 140
Poulsen, L.L. 140, 141
Pourjafar, M. 106, 121
Prastiwi, A. 45

R

Raaijmakers, M. 182
Raboisson, D. 160
Radko, D. 51
Ragažinskienė, O. 153
Ravesloot, L. 101
Rebel, J.M.J. 60, 64, 65
Reese, C.D. 81
Regula-Schüpbach, G. 33
Reimann, E. 108
Reimert, I. 174
Reinhardt, H. 135
Remmelink, G.J. 105, 158
Renaudeau, D. 78
Revskij, D. 198
Rimbach, G. 69
Rodenburg, T.B. 176
Romero-Zúñiga, J.J. 103
Röntgen, M. 154
Roskam, J.L. 126
Rosseel, E. 79
Rothstein, T. 74
Roubos, P. 64
Rovers, M. 87
Rowland, R.R.R. 150
Ruoff, J. 100
Rutten, V.P.M.G. 101

Ruysbergh, E.	63
Rychlik, M.	107

S

Saadat Akhtar, I.	121
Saatkamp, H.W.	124, 126, 175
Saberivand, A.	170
Saborío-Montero, A.	103
Sadri, H.	111
Saiz, A.	88
Sakha, M.	113, 125
Sakkas, P.	132, 142, 152
Šalomskas, A.	153
Samarütel, J.	108
Sander, S.J.	53
Santman-Berends, I.M.G.A.	112, 116, 188, 189
Sarjokari, K.	133
Sasaki, T.	167
Sato, S.	193, 194
Sauerwein, H.	96, 111
Schaeffer, S.	156
Schlederer, F.	183, 191, 199
Schmicke, M.	115
Schokker, D.	60, 64, 65, 76
Schrader, L.	49
Schröder, B.	110, 114
Schuberth, H.J.	198
Schüller, L.K.	84, 86
Schüpbach-Regula, G.	44, 119
Schut, M.L.W.	126
Segers, L.	87
Sejian, V.	80
Sematovica, I.	184
Seppä-Lassila, L.	133
Serao, N.V.L.	150
Shapiev, I.	91
Sierzant, K.	155
Siljander-Rasi, H.	144
Sjöström, K.	181, 192
Slagter, H.	143
Smajlhodzic, F.	48
Smits, M.A.	60, 64, 65
Smolenaars, A.	189
Soede, N.M.	66, 158, 164, 165
Sonck, B.	89
Sordillo, L.M.	95

Soveri, T.	133
Stange, K.	154
Starič, J.	134, 196
Starke, A.	33, 107
Steckeler, P.	169
Stegeman, J.A.	52
Steiner, A.	32, 33, 44
Stewart, G.	152
Stockhofe-Zurwieden, N.	174
Straub, C.	169
Stravakakis, S.	152
Strous, J.E.M.	165
Stygar, A.H.	149
Suetomi, Y.	167
Sullivan, M.L.	80
Sundrum, A.	181, 186

T

Tacher, S.	155
Tasdemir, U.	171
Tedo, G.	69
Ten Wolthuis, A.	36
Thanner, S.	67
Thøfner, I.	140, 141
Tietze, R.	115
Timurkan, M.O.	127
Tiso, N.	153
Topal, O.	138
Torki, M.	65, 76
Tranter, R.B.	148, 186
Tröscher, A.	107, 198
Tsousis, G.	98
Tsukamura, H.	167
Tuchscherer, A.	198
Tuyttens, F.A.M.	38, 89

U

Üffing, B.	53
Urh, C.	96
Ursinus, W.W.	177
Uzochukwu, I.E.	92

V

Vakili, H.	111
Vale, A.	130
Van Beers-Schreurs, H.	132
Vandaele, L.	109

Van Dalen, A.B.J.	42	Viergutz, T.	198
Van Den Borne, J.J.G.C.	132	Visscher, C.	51, 55, 56
Van Den Brand, H.	182	Von Bergen, M.	94
Van Der Aar, P.J.	70, 166	Vrielinck, L.	147
Van Der Beek, S.	190		
Van Der Drift, S.G.A.	112	**W**	
Van Der Eijk, J.A.J.	176	Wagner, T.	98
Van Der Goot, J.A.	52	Wallgren, T.	180
Van Der Peet, C.M.C.	177	Wang, W.	75
Van Der Peet, G.F.V.	177	Watanabe, Y.	193
Van Der Peet-Schwering, C.M.C.	66, 132, 165	Wealleans, A.	62
Van Der Poel, W.H.M.	163	Weaver, S.	93
Van Der Voort, M.	122	Weber, C.	107, 198
Van Der Vorst, Y.	34	Wehrend, A.	183
Van De Ven, L.F.J.	182	Werkman, M.	163
Van Dixhoorn, I.D.E.	174	Westin, R.	180
Van Doorn, D.	200	Wiedemann, S.	98
Van Eetvelde, M.	109	Wilkens, M.R.	110, 114
Van Emous, R.A.	65	Willet, A.	48
Van Engelen, E.	36, 43	Witte, M.	53
Van Essen-Zandbergen, A.	52	Witteveen, G.	188
Van Ginneken, C.	75	Wolfs, E.	182
Van Harn, J.	47	Worm, H.	34
Van Hoeij, R.J.	97, 102, 120		
Van Knegsel, A.T.M.	97, 102, 104, 105, 117, 120, 158	**X**	
		Xu, W.	120
Van Krimpen, M.M.	65, 76		
Van Laer, E.	89	**Y**	
Van Limbergen, T.	147	Yanmaz, L.	45
Van Nieuwamerongen, S.E.	66, 165	Yano, H.	193
Van Noten, N.	75	Yilmazbas-Mecitoglu, G.	171
Van Oostrum, M.	70	Yin, T.	178
Van Riet, M.	38		
Van Saun, R.J.	82, 136, 162	**Z**	
Van Schaik, G.	34, 116, 189	Zamokas, G.	168
Van Staaveren, N.	129, 130	Zarei, M.H.	121
Vargas-Leitón, B.	103	Zavadilová, L.	128
Vastenhouw, S.A.	64, 65	Žilaitis, V.	168
Veissier, I.	89	Zoet, L.	182
Velarde, A.	186	Zolnere, E.	68
Veldman, K.T.	52		
Velge, P.	156		
Velthuis, A.	36, 188		
Vergauwen, H.	75		
Verspohl, J.	53		
Vervoort, J.J.M.	120		
Verwer, C.	48		